"Fleshly lusts…wage war against the s[…] passions pose the deadliest kind of sp[…] The battle we face against such temp[…] half-heartedly. Emeal "E.Z." Zwayne gives an urgent and inspiring call to arms for men in the throes of temptation—and he rightly sounds the trumpet without any hint of uncertainty. If you are not winning the war against carnal lusts, read *Fight Like a Man*. Every man needs the help this excellent book offers.

Dr. John MacArthur, senior pastor of Grace Community Church

If God made men to fight, the most essential battles are won not by the strongest or most experienced but by those warriors who have clean hands and a pure heart. They're not perfect but purehearted like David. If you want to slay the giant of lust in your youth or kill the monster of sexual shame once and for all or finally become "a man after God's own heart," read *Fight Like a Man*. It's an eye-opening and transformational book! Like a powerful Jedi Master, Emeal "E.Z." Zwayne shares practical and precise biblical principles that will teach you how to put to death the evil deeds of darkness and grow strong in your abilities as a mighty man of faith, integrity, and courage.

Kirk Cameron, actor and producer

I believe beyond any doubt that the Bible has proven to be more relevant than tomorrow's breaking news. The Word of God holds the answers to every situation of life. Emeal "E.Z." Zwayne has masterfully woven together profound insights, practical guidance, and unwavering biblical truth to illuminate the often-challenging journey toward sexual purity. Grounded in the timeless teachings of Scripture, this publication serves as a beacon of hope and a road map for those seeking to live a life in accordance with God's design.

Jack Hibbs, senior pastor of Calvary Chapel Chino Hills

If you look up the word *wisdom* in the dictionary, you'll see a picture of Emeal "E.Z." Zwayne. Whenever I need godly wisdom (and it's often), he is my go-to person. As you read *Fight Like a Man*, which is unquestionably one of the most powerful books of its kind, you also will partake in the riches of his godly discernment. This insightful book is written from a passionate conviction that is rooted in personal experience and in Scripture. It's a practical battle plan for this never-ending war that rages in the soul of every man. As you soak in its truths, they will strengthen you in your walk and help you guard yourself from the sharp and fiery darts of the Evil One.

Ray Comfort, founder and CEO of Living Waters

Sadly, today's males who are voyeuristically seeking to feel like men while staring into their electronic screens are in fact stripping away their masculinity one click and fantasy at a time. E.Z.'s insightful and forthright approach to tackling the variety of expressions of this private struggle with illicit lusts provides the biblical light and spiritual equipment for men to fight this good fight of faith in their sanctification. Read this book and make sure it is utilized far and wide to help today's Christian males become real men.

Dr. Mike Fabarez, senior pastor of Compass Bible Church

This book is a weapon that should hang on every man's spiritual wall. With his inimitable passion and creative flare, E.Z. provides a tremendous resource to battle the life-destroying sins of lust, pornography, and adultery. Through heartfelt narratives and practical insights, this book emphasizes the paramount importance of purity and guides readers toward building meaningful, lasting, and God-honoring relationships.

Dr. Tony Wood, pastor-teacher of Mission Bible Church

The title of this book alone is enough to make every feminist furious… and every demon tremble. *Fight Like a Man* is the book you need to defeat the enemy of pornography because it is loaded with one weapon sufficient for victory: the Word of God. Emeal "E.Z." Zwayne bleeds Bible, and that is precisely what you need to mortify the deeds of the flesh. You don't need a feather duster as you engage in your battle against porn. You need weapons of mass destruction. *Fight Like a Man* will arm you to wage war and finally have victory over the sin that so entangles you.

Todd Friel, host of *Wretched Radio* and *Wretched TV*

Lust breeds despair—but the gospel produces hope. That's the truth that pulses like an uncontained electrical current through this biblical, spiritual, and, dare I say, fun book from Emeal "E.Z." Zwayne. E.Z.'s mind is so lively that he offers us men numerous thought devices and helpful mnemonics by which to kill sin and glorify Christ. Here is a book we have been waiting for and greatly needing. It will strengthen us to say a joyful yes to Jesus but a firm NOPE to temptation.

Dr. Owen Strachan, provost and research professor of theology at Grace Bible Theological Seminary

Scripture promises, "No temptation has overtaken you but such as is common to man" (1 Corinthians 10:13 NASB1995). Nevertheless, certain temptations assault men today with a frequency and ferocity that our ancestors did not face. The internet and other media relentlessly push vivid content designed only to appeal to the lust of the flesh and the lust of the eyes. The devil, the world, and our own carnal desires collude to try to gain mastery over us and hold us under sin's power. This is where spiritual warfare is most real and most dangerous. Men today more than ever need to take a militant stance against these temptations, armed with the full panoply of spiritual armor. We *must* be ruthlessly aggressive in the war against sin—not merely to tame or manage it but to mortify it completely. E.Z. understands the urgency of this need, and he has written this remarkably practical, helpful, and encouraging call to arms for men under siege.

Phil Johnson, executive director of Grace to You

Sin is sin, right? All sin is exceedingly sinful, but sexual sin is singled out in Scripture as particularly pernicious and injurious. My friend Emeal "E.Z." Zwayne has taken this tough issue head on. *Fight Like a Man* is not only gospel centered and saturated with Scripture; it is also a truly enjoyable and engaging read. It is very relatable. E.Z. writes in such a way that you will not only be brought face-to-face with the sobering dangers of this deadly sin but also be encouraged to fight this battle with the very real hope and power found in the gospel. This book is a page-turner and one I promise you will be glad you have read. I have many conversations with and receive many emails from men who confess to me that lust is a besetting sin with which they constantly battle and fear they will never gain victory. It will be my joy to recommend this book to them, and it is my joy to enthusiastically recommend it to you.

Justin Peters, president of Justin Peters Ministries

It is hard to stay clean in a coal mine, and it is hard "to keep oneself unspotted from the world" (James 1:27). But the book you hold in your hand is a bar of biblical soap that will help wash off the dirt and grime of sexual temptation and sin in a man's life. Here is a book that comes clean on the need for men to fight for their purity and how to do it and how to do it victoriously in Christ. Victory in the battle for purity will cost, but defeat costs more so. As E.Z.'s pastor, I wholeheartedly endorse the message of this book and its author.

Philip De Courcy, pastor of Kindred Community Church and teacher on the *Know the Truth* radio program

FIGHT

A BOLD, BIBLICAL BATTLE PLAN

LIKE A

FOR PERSONAL PURITY

MAN

EMEAL "E.Z." ZWAYNE

BroadStreet
PUBLISHING

BroadStreet Publishing® Group, LLC
Savage, Minnesota, USA
BroadStreetPublishing.com

Fight Like a Man: A Bold, Biblical Battle Plan for Personal Purity
Copyright © 2024 Emeal Zwayne

9781424568550 (softcover)
9781424568567 (ebook)

All rights reserved. No part of this book may be reproduced in any
form, except for brief quotations in printed reviews, without permission
in writing from the publisher.

Unless otherwise indicated, all Scripture quotations are taken from
the New King James Version® (NKJV). Copyright © 1982 by Thomas
Nelson. Used by permission. All rights reserved. Scripture quotations
marked ESV are taken from the ESV® Bible (The Holy Bible, English
Standard Version®). Copyright © 2001 by Crossway, a publishing
ministry of Good News Publishers. Used by permission. All rights
reserved. Scripture quotations marked NASB are taken from the New
American Standard Bible® (NASB). Copyright © 1960, 1962, 1963,
1968, 1971, 1972, 1973, 1975, 1977, 1995, 2020 by The Lockman
Foundation. Used by permission. www.Lockman.org. Scripture
quotations marked NASB1995 are taken from the New American
Standard Bible® (NASB). Copyright © 1960, 1962, 1963, 1968, 1971,
1972, 1973, 1975, 1977, 1995 by The Lockman Foundation. Used by
permission. www.Lockman.org. Scripture quotations marked KJV are
taken from the King James Version of the Bible, public domain.

Cover and interior by Garborg Design Works | garborgdesign.com

Printed in China

24 25 26 27 28 5 4 3 2 1

To my precious wife, Rachel—
"You excel them all" (Proverbs 31:29).

To my darling daughters, Julia, Summer, and Kylie,
who are lovelier than the daughters of Job.

To my beloved sons, Luke and Danny, and my dear son-in-law,
Matthias—all great men of valor, even mightier than
the mighty men of David, alongside whom I'm honored to fight.

To my late father and mother, Francis and Rosette,
who gave me life, love, and guidance.

To my siblings, Frank, Mona, Nadia, and Nada,
who are the best brother and sisters ever.

To my mother-in-law, Sue, whose kindness and care
have enriched my life.

To my father-in-law, my boss, my mentor, my friend, and the most
faithful man of God I've ever known, Ray Comfort. Only eternity will
reveal the incalculable impact you've had on my life.

To my Lord and Savior Jesus Christ—
without whom I am nothing.

CONTENTS

FOREWORD

We live at a time when there is a great lack of godly male leadership in the world. God gave men the role of being influential leaders in every sphere of society, but so many men have shirked this important responsibility. And Scripture warns us that because of our sin nature, men will not want to be leaders as they should be.

Also, as descendants of Adam, we have a sin nature that wants to be master over our lives. In this fallen world we live in, it is so easy for men to let sin master them and allow destructive sinful desires to rule over them, thus destroying their ability to be the godly leaders they've been called to be.

In a masterful way, my good friend Emeal Zwayne, or "E.Z." as he is called, deals head-on with the issues of male leadership and sexual sin that so need to be addressed in our church culture.

It's "no holds barred" for E.Z. as he challenges men concerning sexual purity. The statistics of men addicted to pornography and other sexual sins, even in the church, are horrific. But E.Z. doesn't just give statistics and his opinions (though he does include engaging stories from his family and travels). I love the way he begins by building his entire case on God's Word, beginning in Genesis. Genesis 1–11 is the foundation for everything, for the rest of the Bible, for a truly Christian worldview, and for all doctrine. That is the only place to start to build the correct worldview for roles and behavior.

Remember, "The word of God is living and active, sharper than any two-edged sword, piercing to the division of soul and of spirit, of joints and of marrow, and discerning the thoughts and intentions of the heart" (Hebrews 4:12 ESV). E.Z. uses God's Word to challenge men concerning their thoughts and behavior. Warning: this book is extremely convicting.

Men can have victory in the area of sexual purity by not letting this sin become master over them. They can overcome any temptation in Christ. "No temptation has overtaken you except such as is common to man; but God is faithful, who will not allow you to be tempted beyond what you are able, but with the temptation will also make the way of escape, that you may be able to bear it" (1 Corinthians 10:13 NKJV). That's why we all need to judge our behavior and thoughts against the absolute authority of God's Word. And E.Z. challenges men to do just that.

It's time for Christian men to rise up and be real men—men as God intended men to be.

I've heard marketing for tours of the Holy Land say that after you visit Israel, "you'll never be the same." Men, read this book, and I guarantee you will never be the same.

Ken Ham

Founder and CEO of Answers in Genesis, the Creation Museum, and the Ark Encounter

PREFACE

Necessity and passion. Critics have rightly said that these two elements must be present for any book to reach its highest potential and achieve its greatest impact. I can't think of a time in the annals of human history when there was a greater necessity for addressing the topic of sexual purity. And the thought of liberating men from bondage to sexual sin infuses this writer with more passion than words could ever express.

There's no question that sexual immorality has reigned supreme across the generations since Adam and Eve's fall in the garden of Eden. However, man's ever-deepening plunge into depravity over many millennia and the aid that modern technologies provide for the enhancement of carnal pleasures have combined to create a climate of perversion unlike anything this planet has seen since its creation.

It may be safe to say that authors within the span of multiple generations have sufficiently covered certain topics and that new books dealing with the same subject matter would be painfully redundant. But I would contend that the issue of sexual purity is a rare exception in this regard—and this is true for two main reasons. First, owing to the insidious, pervasive, and overtly destructive nature of sexual immorality, enough books could never be written to help men find victory in this arena. Secondly, there is an unfortunate and glaring dearth of books written on this topic from a soundly biblical perspective.

The tragic and inevitable by-product of such an atmosphere is a debilitating desensitization to the seriousness of sexual sin. A worldly "Christianity" that has sold its soul to this godless age for the sake of acceptance, relevance, and ease has partly facilitated this desensitization. Tragically, this confluence of elements has left the men of this era in a very precarious predicament. And the church's abdication of duty has deprived men of the correction, exhortation, guidance, and scriptural truth that they so desperately need.

I know—this all sounds quite dismal, doesn't it? But it's against the stifling darkness of such bleak backdrops that the glorious gospel shines brightest. The gospel of Christ is far more than an instrument through

11

which souls are saved. It's also the inexhaustible source and ever-flowing fountain of spiritual riches that supplies the redeemed with every necessary component for developing and nurturing a God-oriented life. So it's by no coincidence that this book is thoroughly gospel-centric, and it's expressly because of the hope that the gospel lavishly supplies that I've written it. What a glorious hope that is! Christ became sin for sinners so that He can impute His spotless righteousness to their account (Romans 5:21). He then takes those who stand in that perfect righteousness and begins to sanctify them day by day as He progressively conforms them into the image of Christ (Hebrews 10:14; Romans 8:29).

When the gospel's power is fully unleashed, it quickens a complacent church to proclaim the truth to its people, reverses the curse of desensitization to sin, and tenderly draws believers toward genuine repentance. This, after all, is what God designed His glorious gospel of grace to do: "The grace of God that brings salvation has appeared to all men, teaching us that, denying ungodliness and worldly lusts, we should live soberly, righteously, and godly in the present age" (Titus 2:11–12).

I hope this liberating and transforming gospel grace will activate a zeal for righteousness in every man who reads this book. I pray that the awareness that they are not their own but were bought with the precious, priceless blood of Christ will cause them to flee sexual immorality and to glorify God with their body and spirit, which belong to Him (1 Corinthians 6:18–20).

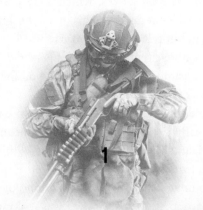

THE THEATER OF WAR

SETTING THE STAGE

A Man Forged in Fire

As exploding grenades and mortar bombs lit up the night sky on the island of Guadalcanal, the beleaguered warriors from First Battalion, Seventh Marines were in for the fight of their lives. Stranded in the South Pacific on one of the more than nine hundred islands that make up Solomon Islands, the small US contingent of World War II combatants was under siege by three thousand Japanese troops. Outnumbered and outgunned, the marines bravely held their ground and repelled wave after wave of enemy fighters. Just when it seemed like they were turning the tide, incoming fire damaged and disabled one of the combat crews' main artillery. Defying every instinct of self-preservation, the commanding officer, Gunnery Sergeant John Basilone, did the unthinkable. Exposing himself to flying bullets and hidden enemies attacking at random, he ran six hundred feet to the defunct pit while carrying close to one hundred pounds of weapons and ammunition. Back and forth he went between his foxhole and that of his comrades, providing supplies and aid while simultaneously picking off opposing soldiers with nothing but a pistol in hand.

Having lost his special gloves, which were necessary protection from the searing heat generated by his machine gun, Basilone sustained burns from holding it barehanded. He was credited with killing thirty-eight enemies himself, and as one of his fellow marines, Nash W. Phillips, reported, "Basilone had a machine gun on the go for three days and nights without sleep, rest, or food."[1]

After the battalion victoriously survived the battle, Phillips was being treated for his injuries when the sergeant came in to check on him. "He was barefooted, and his eyes were red as fire," Phillips recalled. "His face was dirty black from gunfire and lack of sleep. His shirt sleeves were rolled up to his shoulders. He had a .45 tucked into the waistband of his trousers. He'd just dropped by to see how I was making out; me and the others in the section. I'll never forget him."[2]

After receiving the Congressional Medal of Honor, John Basilone was given the opportunity to spend the rest of the war in the safety of Washington, DC. John refused and instead returned to the heat of battle. In his final act of courage, bravery, and selflessness, he stormed the shores of Iwo Jima on February 19, 1945. While Sergeant Basilone's life ended there, the ripples created by his sacrificial heroism continue to touch lives around the world to this day.[3]

I wonder how John Basilone's story strikes you. Does his legendary altruism rouse a sense of admiration in your heart? Does his harrowing sacrifice evoke terror in the core of your being as you imagine yourself running across the raging battlefield in his boots? Is it possible that perhaps—in a sort of defining moment—it inspires a longing in you to follow in his footsteps as you fight your way through the biggest war of all—the one we call life?

A Man-to-Man Talk about Real Manhood

I wish you and I were sitting together at my favorite coffee shop right now. It's a rustic kind of place. A mixture of used bricks, rough wood, metal fixtures, and distressed concrete floors makes it the perfect setting for a good old-fashioned, man-to-man talk. I would look you straight in

1   John Simkins, "Valor Friday: The Legend of John Basilone," *Marine Corps Times*, June 29, 2018, https://www.marinecorpstimes.com.
2   Simkins, "Valor Friday."
3   Simkins, "Valor Friday."

the eye and ask you a fundamental question, the kind of question that every man should be asked—or at least the one that every man should be asking himself: *What defines a real man?*

Does this bring back memories of a US Supreme Court nominee saying no after a senator asked her if she could define the word *woman*? You and I both know that the world has completely lost its perspective on all things related to gender. When so-called influencers tell us that "men" can menstruate and conceive babies and when expectant mothers are now called "birthing persons" who have the ability to "chest feed," you know that, Houston, we've got far more than just a problem. We've got an epic catastrophe on our hands. At a time when those who occupy the highest and most respectable echelons of society are publicly declaring that they can't define what a man or a woman is, is it any wonder that men are losing sight of what it really means to be a man?

What I'm about to say has become so taboo in our upside-down world that those who would dare even to whisper this sort of thing are instantly shunned, cast out, and "canceled" as immoral dregs by the self-appointed guardians of this godless age. For the pleasure of my Savior and out of love for others, I'll gladly endure that ill-treatment—and much worse. Here goes! Note this well: John Basilone's life bears the marks of real manhood.

Before you tune out here, let me put some meat on those bones. Sergeant Basilone's masculinity was not determined by the fact that he was a marine, nor was it because he was physically tough or adept at combat. It was not even because he might have been athletic, had a thick beard, or spoke in a deep voice. A male can be all those things and still not act like a real man. And by the same token, Basilone could have been none of those things and still have been the manliest of men.

Our war hero's life bears the marks of real manhood because real men demonstrate character, courage, commitment, conviction, devotion, and loyalty. And what's more, they're willing to sacrifice for the sake of others and for causes greater than themselves. Most importantly, real men are willing to fight for what's right, and they do so in the energy and spirit of those indispensable attributes I just highlighted. Pastor and author Robert Lewis reinforces and aptly articulates what I'm trying to convey:

What is a real man?…A real man is one who:
- rejects passivity
- accepts responsibility
- leads courageously
- expects the greater reward…God's reward.

This manhood vision desperately needs to be proclaimed throughout our society.[4]

What Type of Warrior Are You?

So back to that other kind of war that I mentioned. While a tiny percentage of the world's men will ever traipse across the theater of conventional warfare, every man born of a woman—and that's *every* man—enters this world as an enlisted private in the inescapable war of life. While that automatic designation, by default, includes the title of warrior, a man's chosen conduct in that capacity will determine the qualifying adjective that precedes that inherited title. Certain men choose irresponsibility and go AWOL. Others opt to become traitors and consort with the enemy. Some pick the pathway of faintheartedness and raise the white flag of surrender. And then you have the men of mediocrity—the ones who do the absolute minimum to get by and barely survive. These are the irresponsible, traitorous, cowardly, and mediocre warriors. But a few determine to tread the road less traveled and become the faithful, honorable, relentless, dedicated, and victorious warriors.

Within the broader context of the war of life, there is a sort of sub-war that every man finds himself engulfed in. It typically starts at the onset of puberty and fluctuates in intensity across the varying seasons of adulthood, even into the senior years. I'm obviously talking about the war of sexual temptations.

It would be silly to ask you which type of warrior you want to be in this relentless war. Which God-fearing man would ever seriously say, *Oh, I most certainly want to be an irresponsible, traitorous, cowardly, and mediocre warrior in the war of sexual temptations?* Chances are that most of the men reading this book will have, by now, crossed over the

4   Robert Lewis, *Raising a Modern-Day Knight: A Father's Role in Guiding His Son to Authentic Manhood* (Carol Stream, IL: Tyndale House Publishers, 2007), 60–61.

threshold of puberty. This means that you, my friend, have already made your warrior debut. So instead of asking you what type of warrior you would like to be, it's better to ask what type of warrior you have been in your various battles thus far.

Hope for the Weary

I realize at this point that the thought of quietly putting this book to rest may seem very appealing to you. Perhaps you've failed miserably with one stumble into sexual sin after another. Your list may include pornography or masturbation. Maybe you've gone as far as fornication or adultery. It could even be a combination of some or all those things. And it's also possible that you can honestly say that your only struggle in the sexual realm has been with the sin of proactively lusting after women in your heart. This could be through images of clothed women (whether in skimpy swimwear or other immodest apparel) that you've searched out or have come across online and via other mediums. Or maybe your main battle has entailed lusting after women you've seen in public or that you've conjured up in your imagination.

No matter how big or prolonged or shameful your sexual sins have been, an overwhelming abundance of hope is available to you in the inexhaustible love and grace of God. The glorious gospel, secured by the death and resurrection of Christ, not only redeems and regenerates but also enables transformative change as it empowers you in ways you may never have thought possible.

In *Finally Free*—one of the most insightful and practical books written on the subject of sexual purity—Heath Lambert beautifully extoled the hope we have in Christ with these powerful words:

> There is no porn user so enslaved that Jesus cannot set him
> or her free. There is no struggle for purity so intense that
> Jesus' grace cannot win the battle. There is no consequence
> so steep that Jesus' power cannot carry you through. Jesus'
> grace to change you is stronger than pornography's power
> to destroy you. Jesus' grace is stronger than your own
> desires to watch sex. While there is no hope for you in

looking at pornography, there is all the hope in the universe when you look to God and His grace.[5]

Despite how much you may have failed thus far in your calling to be a faithful, honorable, relentless, dedicated, and victorious warrior, your magnificent Redeemer has made provision for you to change the trend and begin fighting like a man.

But unfortunately, real men are in short supply today. Cultural theologian P. Andrew Sandlin couldn't have said it better: "One of the most tragic cultural shifts of the U.S. in the last quarter century is the loss of rugged manliness. In my experience, most young men, including young Christian men, suffer from laziness; lack of ambition; obsession with cheap entertainment; a void of chivalry or protection of women; and a whiny, self-centered, non-risktaking disposition."[6]

And yet, God's Word exhorts us to pursue a higher standard—the standard of real manhood. "Be watchful, stand firm in the faith, act like men, be strong" (1 Corinthians 16:13 ESV).

In his exposition of this verse, Dr. John MacArthur said the following about what it means to act like a man:

"Act like men" essentially means to conduct one's self in a courageous way...

Courage is the stock-in-trade of a man: courage in the face of danger, courage in the face of temptation... There's nothing more manly than a man with consummate conviction, courage, and endurance, who is marked by love. That's a man—not weak, not vacillating, not fearful; and loving.

Real men face life with this kind of fortitude. They're watchful of the dangers around them. They're alert. They're protectors of their wives and children, and of their friends and all the people over whom they have influence.[7]

5   Heath Lambert, *Finally Free: Fighting for Purity with the Power of Grace* (Grand Rapids, MI: Zondervan, 2013), 28.
6   P. Andrew Sandlin, "One of the most tragic cultural shifts of the U.S.," Facebook, July 30, 2021, https://www.facebook.com.
7   John MacArthur, "Act Like Men," Grace to You, June 21, 2020, https://www.gty.org.

Are you willing to stand with that kind of fortitude and fight like a man, my brother? Will you determine to stand and be counted? Will you exert every ounce of energy within you to battle through your war of sexual temptations in the same fashion that John Basilone battled his way through World War II? Will you demonstrate character, courage, commitment, conviction, devotion, and loyalty? Will you sacrifice for the sake of others—like your wife, your children, your grandchildren, your parents, your siblings, your friends, your church family, the young people who look up to you as an example, and the older people who have invested their lives in you? And will you lay down your life, through death to self, for causes greater than yourself—like the testimony of the gospel and the glory of God?

A Battle Plan for Your Battle

Let's not be self-deceived about the seriousness and intensity of this war. It's easy for us to psych ourselves up and get inspired by a rousing story like John Basilone's. But as I'm sure you've learned from life by now, feelings of inspiration come and go. It's one thing to envision ourselves doing something with great gusto and enthusiasm. But when the rubber meets the road, it's an entirely different matter.

Can you relate? If you're a man with red blood flowing through your veins and you've never shouted out words such as, "I feel like I'm about to go crazy!" or at least belted them out in the echoey corridors of your exasperated mind, perhaps an emergency pulse check is in order. And while you may have used those words in any number of circumstances, you and I both know that they were never infused with more passion, intensity, and frustration than when you've unleashed them in the context of a struggle with sexual temptations.

It's often been said that there's no force on earth more powerful than the sex drive. There are days when every man has felt like his sex drive could give nuclear energy a run for its money. Though it's true that the overwhelming majority of men at some time find themselves under the sway of sexual urges, this struggle bears an altogether different dynamic for the Christian man. While the unbeliever is a helpless slave to sin and typically exerts no resistance against its dictates, the believer is a slave to Christ and, therefore, finds himself constantly fighting against sexual urges out of a genuine desire to please the Master.

As the battle for sexual purity rages hot in the sincerest and most committed of Christ's servants, many grow exasperated, disheartened, and disillusioned when trying to find a pathway to victory. Some of this is due to misunderstanding the nature of the struggle itself. In other cases, it's because the Christian does not realize that he has received all things that pertain to life and godliness (2 Peter 1:3), which includes victory over sexual temptations. But one element that many men often overlook is the fact that they don't have a comprehensive and gospel-centered battle plan that integrates the fear of God and dynamic spiritual discipline with a biblical understanding of the fallen nature of this world and the spiritual resources available to them in Christ.

A soldier who runs out onto a military battlefield clad in a bathrobe and fluffy slippers with "champagne wishes and caviar dreams" will quickly realize that he really has a death wish and a nightmare on his hands. You're self-deluded if you think that you're on a luxury yacht cruising toward a resort in Bora-Bora when, in reality, you're on a Higgins boat heading for the shores of John Basilone's Guadalcanal. Both disillusion and demise will be the inevitable outcome because, let's face it, vacationers aren't looking to fight or to carry out battle plans; they're fixin' to feast and frolic.

A wartime mentality is hard to cultivate when we live in an atmosphere of ease and luxury—with overwhelming distractions and allurements constantly enticing us to relax, kick up our feet, and coast. The war that rages about us is an invisible one, and this is where the deception lies. While we feel the tension of spiritual battle in the heat of sexual temptation, we don't really sense it very keenly at other times—and this is the very thing that fosters and perpetuates the deceptive illusion, leading us to become complacent and live out most of our days with a peacetime mentality. Then, when the battle suddenly becomes apparent to us, we scramble to fight like an equipped soldier, though we have done nothing whatsoever to adequately equip ourselves.

But before the spiritual battle has reached the boiling point of intense sexual temptation, a thousand other fierce clashes and skirmishes are being waged against our souls—at times directly, at other times behind the scenes—and we cannot let our guard down or turn our back on the Enemy for even one second. Ephesians reminds us of the invisible nature of the warfare that I just referenced, making it clear that we don't wrestle against flesh and blood; our battle is a spiritual one. And our armor and weaponry are invisible and spiritual as well (Ephesians 6:10–17).

This sobering exhortation by Charles H. Spurgeon is worthy of note: "If you will tell me when God permits a Christian to lay aside his armour, I will tell you when Satan has left off temptation. Like the old knights in war time, we must sleep with helmet and breastplate buckled on, for the arch-deceiver will seize our first unguarded hour to make us his prey. The Lord keep us watchful in all seasons, and give us a final escape from the jaw of the lion and the paw of the bear."[8]

To help you further grasp the indispensable necessity of this kind of posture and mindset for every Christian man, focus on these eye-opening words from *Passions of the Heart*, Dr. John Street's exemplary and authoritative work on the subject of sexual purity:

> You must go to battle against sexual lust with the attitude of a soldier—but a soldier who recognizes his own inability to secure a victory. As a soldier, you must be willing to die to self to gain final freedom from sexual slavery. Only then will you realize the transforming grace of Jesus Christ that will bring the final conquest. In the meantime, you are in this battle, waging war against the flesh on the battlefield of the heart. The war is tough because the enemy is often varied, layered, and constantly reproducing. The enemy also knows the territory.[9]

Preventative Preparedness

Remember that war doesn't just involve direct confrontation on the battlefield. That's the typical culmination of the grander scheme of war. Every wise nation that has enemies, just like every wise man who has

---

8   Charles H. Spurgeon, "February 20, Evening," in *Morning and Evening*, accessed August 30, 2020, https://www.biblegateway.com.
9   John D. Street, *Passions of the Heart: Biblical Counsel for Stubborn Sexual Sins* (Phillipsburg, NJ: P&R Publishing, 2019), 210.

spiritual foes seeking to destroy him in the war of sexual temptations, will do everything necessary to avert a direct attack by those who seek to destroy it.

We might think that strong national security is the possession of a sovereign state that maintains overwhelming military might. This, of course, is true but not for the reasons that may seem immediately apparent. We subconsciously conclude that this type of security exists because a particular nation constantly uses its robust military capabilities to directly war against other countries, thus vanquishing them and rendering them a nonthreat. But that's often not the case. In many instances, the strong security of a particular nation is a reality because most other nations would never dare attack it on the battlefield. This is specifically due to what I call its extreme *preventative preparedness*. This includes hyperorganizing, advanced and rigorous training, amassing devastating and state-of-the-art weaponry, and implementing superior defense capabilities, not to mention forming strong alliances with other powerful nations that would immediately come to its defense. This kind of provident, preventative preparedness minimizes such a nation's need to unleash its military might. Simply, as I stated already, other nations wouldn't dare attack it in a conventional way. This is what many military leaders call *peace through strength*. And in the rare event that some misguided regime would be foolhardy enough to launch an assault against such a nation, they would undoubtedly rue the day.

It's in this spirit, as it relates to one of our main enemies (and principally applies to the rest), that Scripture reminds us to "submit to God. Resist the devil and he will flee from you. Draw near to God and He will draw near to you" (James 4:7–8).

Once again, Charles H. Spurgeon captured this well:

> Satan does not often attack a Christian who is living near
> to God. It is when the Christian departs from his God,
> becomes spiritually starved, and endeavours to feed on
> vanities, that the devil discovers his vantage hour. He may
> sometimes stand foot to foot with the child of God who
> is active in his Master's service, but the battle is gener-
> ally short: he who slips as he goes down into the Valley

of Humiliation, every time he takes a false step invites Apollyon to assail him.[10]

Know Your Enemies

In the war of sexual temptations, you have three ruthless enemies who are bent on your destruction. Knowing who they are and understanding the lethal strategies they have formulated against you is a foundational step toward building up the type of preventative preparedness that will neutralize them and give you victory in your quest for sexual purity as you fight like a man. This book aims to present you with that knowledge, provide you with the necessary tools to cultivate that preparedness, and, through inspiration and encouragement from God's Word and the truth of the gospel of grace, help propel you toward that victory.

---

10   Charles H. Spurgeon, "June 13, Evening," in *Morning and Evening*, accessed August 30, 2023, https://www.biblegateway.com.

PART 1

THE DEVIL

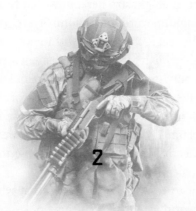

2

PUBLIC ENEMY NUMBER ONE

What Would It Be Like If...?

One of my favorite pastimes is imagining how different a particular element in life would be if a specific component were removed from it. What would our productivity be like if we never had to sleep? What would eating be like if we didn't have taste buds? What would walking around be like if we didn't have gravity? What would the Three Stooges be like if they didn't have Curly? Well, I guess there's no imagination needed there—we all know that tragic outcome. But can you imagine what our existence would be like without any enemies in it? No one looking to deceive us, defraud us, use us, abuse us, attack us, destroy us. That would certainly be a sweet foretaste of heaven. And Scripture promises that one day our Savior will destroy every single enemy: "He must reign till He has put all enemies under His feet. The last enemy that will be destroyed is death" (1 Corinthians 15:25–26).

But that day has not yet arrived. Our adversaries in this world abound. They're alive and well and thriving, constantly seeking to do us much harm. And we unquestionably have no enemies more brutal and pernicious than the three that seek to lead us toward the slaughter of sexual sin: the devil, the flesh, and the world.

It's important to emphasize here, however, that the devil and the world are, in the insightful words of Dr. John Street, "outward adversaries of opportunity."[1] The real archenemy is within; it's the flesh—that fallen, sinful nature that gives birth to what the apostle James called "desires for pleasure" (4:1). It's our "innate lust," which, again, issues forth from the flesh and makes "allies" with the devil and the world.[2] Dr. Street wisely reminded us, "*Man* is fully responsible for his lapse into immoral cravings; the cause of blame is deep within. Satan and the world provide the occasion, but the effectiveness of their temptation is totally dependent on the condition and receptivity of your heart."[3]

It's important to remember, therefore, that whenever I reference the devil and the world as enemies in this book, you should view this designation through the lenses of this broader context.

With this in mind, the first fiendish foe we will examine is the devil. While most Christians are familiar with what Jesus said about Satan's nature, I'm amazed by how often we still fall victim to his insidious machinations. Based on our clear understanding of who he is, we would expect to have more victory over him than we typically do. Instead, we find ourselves falling prey to the thoughts he plants in our heads, the temptations he dangles in front of us, and the stumbling blocks he puts in our way.

Liar, Liar

Imagine personally knowing someone who is reputed to be a pathological liar, someone for whom lying seems to come as naturally as breathing. I'm referring to the type of person about whom others warn, "You can't believe a word they say." A bloke whose honker would make Pinocchio's look like Voldemort's nose. If that individual told you something that contradicted important information that your earthly father communicated to you—your father, who personifies integrity and who never once lied to you—would you entertain the words of Mr. Pants-on-Fire for even a nanosecond?

---

1   John D. Street, *Passions of the Heart: Biblical Counsel for Stubborn Sexual Sins* (Phillipsburg, NJ: P&R Publishing, 2019), 63–64.

2   Street, *Passions of the Heart*, 64.

3   Street, *Passions of the Heart*, 62.

In one of His heated exchanges with the religious hypocrites of His day, Jesus highlighted the devil's nature and character for them. He called Satan "a liar and the father of lies" (John 8:44 ESV). He went so far as to say that there is no truth in him and that when he speaks a lie, he speaks from his own resources. This is a direct reference to the devil's nature—meaning that it's impossible for him to speak anything but lies because he's got nothing but lies in him. In other words, it would be as impossible to draw truth from Satan's diabolical lips as it would be to draw flames of fire from a bucket full of ice water in a vacuum-sealed room. This, of course, is hyperbolic. It doesn't literally mean that Satan can never make factually true statements (as there are examples in Scripture when he clearly did), but the thrust is that he thoroughly infuses deception into all his schemes.

Don't Fall for It...Again

And so, the most maniacal, pathological liar in the universe continues accosting the sons of Adam and the daughters of Eve with the same slimy tactic that he used on their parents at the dawn of creation. He's a one-trick pony. We know his name, his game, his claim to fame, yet we continue swallowing his lies—hook, line, and sinker. Proverbs 1:17 says, "Surely, in vain the net is spread in the sight of any bird." In other words, as dumb as birds are (my apologies to bird lovers), if they see you standing there seeking to trap them, they won't come near you and walk into your trap. Unfortunately, we've not only seen Satan standing there seeking to trap us, but we've watched countless people get ensnared in his trap and destroy their lives royally. We ourselves have walked into that same trap more times than we'd like to remember and have the limp to prove it. And yet, we willingly walk ourselves right back into it on a regular basis.

It's fitting that the very next verse in Proverbs goes on to say, "They lie in wait for their own blood, they lurk secretly for their own lives" (1:18). The sad thing is that each time we walk ourselves into Satan's trap, we act as though the outcome will be different from what it was before. Like jumping off a skyscraper is definitely going to give us the power of flight the next time. Insanity! And it's rightly been said that the definition of *insanity* is doing the same thing over and over again and expecting a different result.

In the next chapter, we'll journey back to Eden and replay the infamous scene that plunged the whole of creation into utter ruin. We'll examine the details of the insidious lie that the Serpent of old told God's freshly minted image-bearers, and we'll consider the severity of sin at its very core.

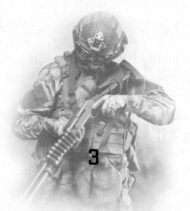

3

THE DEVIL'S "SAME OLD, SAME OLD"

DISCONTENT, DISBELIEF, AND DEIFICATION

Discontent

To Their Hearts' Content

Paradise was sweet for the soon-to-be Papa Adam and Mama Eve. At that point, there weren't any little scream machines waking them up five times in the middle of the night, no terrible-twos temper tantrums to deal with, and no fig leaf diapers to change (ouch). It was like an endless honeymoon—the most epic life imaginable for the newlyweds. Perfect weather. An array of leafy, natural food-producing factories. No marital problems. No health issues. No financial struggles. No meddling in-laws. No dandruff. No taxes. No I-can't-find-anything-in-my-closet-to-wear-today struggles. No belly-button lint. No sorrow, no grief, and no death. And to top it all off, they got to stroll around the garden while living in perfect harmony with the creator of the universe. What more could they ever want? Well, only the one thing they couldn't have, of course.

God spared no creative expenses when He crafted an impeccably suitable world for His perfectly fashioned creatures. He did not overlook a single detail, and He gave them only one prohibition. Just one. And it wasn't the sort of prohibition that eliminated an entire category of enjoyment for them. He didn't say, "You shall not eat," and then insert a period. He didn't create their taste buds and appetites only to deprive them of the pleasure of satisfying them. It's best to let God speak for Himself: "The LORD God commanded the man, saying, 'Of every tree of the garden you may freely eat'" (Genesis 2:16).

Notice that the Lord didn't tell Adam and Eve that they could only eat at certain times or only a limited amount of food at given intervals or that they were only permitted to eat from select trees on specific days. He didn't crack open the door of permissiveness; He blew it off the hinges when He said "of every" and "freely." And He didn't give them bland, tasteless survival food. Here are the details, and there's no devil in them—yet. "Out of the ground the LORD God made every tree grow that is pleasant to the sight and good for food" (v. 9). The trees all looked good. And along with being pleasant to the sight, they also undoubtedly smelled good, tasted good, and *were* good for them.

God didn't just give, but He gave in lavish abundance, providing for His dust-framed handiwork an overflowing supply of riches from His divinely generous heart—a heart bursting with perfect and unquenchable love for them.

And then came the solitary restriction: "Of the tree of the knowledge of good and evil you shall not eat, for in the day that you eat of it you shall surely die" (v. 17).

It was all theirs. Every brook and stream, every lake and ocean, every mountain and desert and valley and prairie, every forest and savanna and plain and jungle. It all belonged to them. God granted them dominion over every square inch of the planet and all that it contained. He made it for their enjoyment and pleasure, placing it all under their authority. God had made this clear from the very start: "God blessed them, and God said to them, 'Be fruitful and multiply; fill the earth and subdue it; have dominion over the fish of the sea, over the birds of the air, and over every living thing that moves on the earth'" (1:28).

The Biggest Dwarf Tree Ever

My jaw nearly hit the ground when I saw it, and I've seen some massive trees in my time, including the famously gargantuan redwoods of California. But this one—this one was undeniably in a league of its own. They call it the árbol del Tule, and, man, was it herculean! It is located in the town of Santa María del Tule, in the Mexican state of Oaxaca. While it measures an impressive 116 feet (35.6 meters) high, its most mind-blowing feature is its girth. With a whopping circumference of 137.8 feet (42 meters), it has been ranked as the widest tree in the world.[1] While I knew I couldn't wrap my arms around it, I tried to wrap my head around its colossal size, but even that didn't work. And if I've piqued your interest enough to look it up, believe me, pictures don't do it justice.

I wonder how the Tree of the Knowledge of Good and Evil would have stacked up against good ole árbol del Tule. The Bible doesn't describe its dimensions, but let's say it was close to the same size. In fact, for argument's sake, let's make it three times bigger—348 feet (106.1 meters) high and 413.4 feet (126 meters) in circumference. How visible would it have been from space? Right—not visible at all. Now contrast it with the scope of the entire planet, the planet over which God gave Adam and Eve complete dominion, and you'll immediately see that it would have been more infinitesimal than a speck of dust in comparison. This gives you an idea of how little God withheld from them when juxtaposed with how much He gave them. And He withheld it for their good.

But when the tempter worked his beguiling witchcraft, Adam and Eve lost sight of every blessing they held in their grasp and became enamored by the one thing they couldn't have. The Bible gives us an example of how an unhealthy preoccupation with what we don't have can cause us to lose appreciation for the blessings that we've received. This then leads to *discontent*—Satan's first tactical temptation toward Eve and one of the most destructive pitfalls man can ever stumble into.

When Everything Isn't Enough

If you've ever read the book of Esther, you would have undoubtedly experienced some sense of amusement after encountering the eccentric villain, Haman—second-in-command over the entire Persian empire.

---

1   Wikipedia, s.v. "Árbol del Tule," last modified May 20, 2023, https://en.m.wikipedia.org.

King Ahasuerus had commanded all his servants to bow before Haman, and Haman's narcissistic preoccupation with garnering homage from all the king's subjects was all-consuming. But Haman had one little problem that came in the form of a man named Mordecai. Because of Mordecai's unwillingness to bow before him, Haman allowed Mordecai to become his undoing. One day, after riding high with joy over what he perceived was a very favorable turn of events for him, something rather peculiar happened:

> Haman went out that day joyful and with a glad heart; but when Haman saw Mordecai in the king's gate, and that he did not stand or tremble before him, he was filled with indignation against Mordecai. Nevertheless Haman restrained himself and went home, and he sent and called for his friends and his wife Zeresh. Then Haman told them of his great riches, the multitude of his children, everything in which the king had promoted him, and how he had advanced him above the officials and servants of the king.
>
> Moreover Haman said, "Besides, Queen Esther invited no one but me to come in with the king to the banquet that she prepared; and tomorrow I am again invited by her, along with the king. Yet all this avails me nothing, so long as I see Mordecai the Jew sitting at the king's gate." (Esther 5:9–13)

Quite astounding, isn't it? Haman wasn't just overflowing with the sorts of blessings that most people could only dream of possessing, but he was keenly aware of them all and how significant they truly were. So much so that he didn't merely ponder them in his mind; he actually gathered an audience around him and highlighted them one by one. Sometimes we might try to excuse ungrateful people by chalking up their ungratefulness to a sense of ignorance regarding how good they really have it. Not so with Haman. He knew, and he knew well. And even against that backdrop of hyperclarity, he dared to utter a line that both confounds and convicts me: "Yet all this avails me nothing."

Did he really say that? *My astonishing wealth, my multiple children, my top-ranking position in the most powerful empire on the planet, and the distinct favor the king and queen have repeatedly given me—all this means nothing to me because this one guy won't bow before me and give me the respect I want.* Unthinkable, right? But before we point a condemning finger at Haman, we would do well to take a long, hard look in the mirror. Of course, we've never articulated such a thing. Most of us wouldn't. We're too prideful to allow ourselves to look that foolish. But is this not what our attitude has screamed from the rooftops time and time again? Is this not what our actions—that, yes, speak much louder than words—have written and painted and sung in a thousand different ways?

Covetousness, the Bible tells us, is idolatry (Colossians 3:5). And idolatry is the root of lust. Dr. John Street put a massive exclamation point on this incontrovertible truth: "At the top of this lineup of deities is covetousness. This idol nourishes all other functional gods. Covetousness is at the root of all sexual sin, and it produces in the heart new and refined idols. Serving and gratifying self is its core expectation."[2]

Keep in mind that lust is not associated solely with sexual sin. We can lust after or covet anything—be it our neighbor's wife, our neighbor's goods, our neighbor's inordinate respect, or anything else imaginable. This idolatrous sin of covetousness, which is fueled by discontent, can lead to a frightening altered state of mind that influences people to do the unthinkable. In Haman's case, it drove him toward genocide; he sought to annihilate every Jew in the entire Persian empire. Seriously? Seeking to destroy an entire people group because one guy refused to bow before you? Insane! But idolatry doesn't operate in the realm of sanity.

The Hypnotizing Shape-Shifter

This is the Father of Lies's primary tactic. He deceives us into believing that all is not right in our little universe until we get that one thing. And once we stare deeply enough into his lie to become hypnotized by it, everything else loses its relevance. We become suspicious of God and begin doubting His good intentions toward us. We despise His overwhelmingly generous blessings, becoming chronically discontent. And we do the unthinkable as we chase after the wind and try to grasp it in our hands.

---

2   John D. Street, *Passions of the Heart: Biblical Counsel for Stubborn Sexual Sins* (Phillipsburg, NJ: P&R Publishing, 2019), 101.

When we finally do obtain that one thing that we were passion-ately lusting after, lust, as Heath Lambert aptly put it, "guarantees that as soon as you possess the object of your longing, you will get a new greedy desire for something more."[3]

Satan's first lie was couched in some shifty sleight-of-hand play with God's words. With this initial ploy, he didn't come out blatantly and say that God said something contrary to what He had actually said. Satan took a slier and subtler approach. After all, Scripture tells us that the devil can disguise himself as an angel of light (2 Corinthians 11:14). He can come across as a pure being with pure motives and intentions—the one who's always there to look out for you and serve your best interests.

So he launched his attack with a question for the woman. He didn't say, "God said such and such," but he asked, "Has God indeed said, 'You shall not eat of every tree of the garden'?" (Genesis 3:1). Notice the insidious tactic the deceiver employed. He didn't focus on the Tree of the Knowledge of Good and Evil. In fact, he didn't even mention it. He planted the seeds of suspicion and discontent by making it seem as though God was egregiously unfair for not allowing the man and woman to eat of *every* single tree in the garden. Never mind that the Lord allowed them to eat of every single tree freely and without limit—*except* for just one—and gave them dominion over the entire planet and everything in it.

Disbelief

The Deceptive Painter and the Tricky Boxer
With the seeds of suspicion and discontent firmly planted in Eve's mind, the Enemy launched his second assault: *disbelief*. This time he unasham-edly contradicted God's clear decree. "You will not surely die" (v. 4). He was meticulously painting the picture. After the first strokes that cast God as an unfair and stingy Father, the Father of Lies now dared to make the Creator out to be a liar.

Think about how many problems would be solved if everyone simply believed everything God said. Isn't disbelief often at the root of our waywardness and rebellion? Instead of taking God at His word and

---

3   Heath Lambert, *Finally Free: Fighting for Purity with the Power of Grace* (Grand Rapids, MI: Zondervan, 2013), 130.

yielding in obedience to Him, we choose to believe demonically inspired lies. By default, we end up scoffing at what the Lord has revealed about the guaranteed consequences of our sinful actions.

This is the epitome of blindness. Satan first introduced this sneaky strategy in Eden, but as Scripture demonstrates, he has continued to employ it in different contexts—and most devastatingly, as it relates to the gospel: "Even if our gospel is veiled, it is veiled to those who are perishing, whose minds the god of this age has blinded, who do not believe, lest the light of the gospel of the glory of Christ, who is the image of God, should shine on them" (2 Corinthians 4:3–4).

Blindness and disbelief—that's his standard one-two combination punch, and Satan is adept at using it in many different contexts. He works his enchanting magic by launching a left jab of deceit to disorient people's eyes and keep them from clearly seeing the significance of what God has revealed. Then he hits them with a jarring right cross of doubt, sending them flying toward the abyss of faithlessness.

Forewarned and Forearmed

Bear in mind the kindness that God demonstrated toward Adam and Eve when He made clear what the outcome would be if they chose to rebel against His unambiguous command. He wasn't obligated to do this. He could have simply highlighted the prohibition and left it at that. But in His divine love, He held nothing back. Yes, as you've heard it said, to be forewarned is to be forearmed. God graciously forewarned His beloved stewards with knowledge so that they would be forearmed with wisdom.

Satan was undoubtedly aware that the foundation of true wisdom is the fear of the Lord (Proverbs 9:10). This type of godly fear has respect, honor, and awe at its very core. Satan knew that for Eve to forsake the way of wisdom and act in a manner contrary to the knowledge that God had revealed to her about the consequences of disobedience, he had to diminish her fear of the Lord. He did this by conjuring up doubts in her mind about her Maker's character. He implied that her Master was not to be trusted because He was a deceiver with no intention—and, by extension, no power—to follow through on His promised judgment. And obviously, a God of such corrupt character wouldn't be worthy of respect, honor, awe, and obedience. So the devil thundered, "You will not

FIGHT LIKE A MAN

surely die," and the woman bought the horrid creature's lie rather than believing the truth of her holy Creator.

Deification

What's in It for Me?

Having shaken and weakened Eve's foundation with his first two bunker busters, the soon-to-be-slithering fiend next pressed the red button and launched his nuclear bomb. He hit Eve with the infamous "What's in it for me?" tactic: *You can gain a great power that God is withholding from you, an immense power that is good for you—wonderful and amazing beyond compare. In fact, Eve, you can be like God.*

Godlikeness. Is it any wonder that Satan would tempt Eve with the very thing that brought about his own downfall? "I will ascend above the heights of the clouds, I will be like the Most High," he said (Isaiah 14:14). And his lie here is compounded by the very fact that he learned, by experience, the impossibility and futility of such a foolish ambition. But what was the shimmering jewel within this temptation of godlikeness that would have flashed with dazzling brilliance before Eve's innocent eyes? Autonomy! And through autonomy, a vain pursuit of attaining ultimate fulfillment through one's own devices. Fully independent of God, the man and woman could make their own call on what is good and evil.

I shuddered as I typed those words because they're devastatingly true and because I've seen them fulfilled in myself every time I've chosen to sin instead of placing myself under the rule of God in obedience to His divine decrees.

Autono-me and You

Is this not indeed the driving force behind every sinful pursuit that every fallen human being has ever undertaken? We want to be free to do what we want despite what God has said is best for us. We may deceive ourselves into thinking that we aren't really saying that we want to be like God simply by choosing to sin, but what else could our actions mean? Amid our rebellious actions, are we saying, "I want to be under the rule of God right now; I want to bow before Him in worship as I yield to His will; I want to deny myself and trust that He knows better than I do;

I want to forget about glorying in my sinful pleasures and live for His glory alone"? If we can concur that this is not what our sinful actions are demonstrating, then we must conclude that they are saying the exact opposite: "I want to be under my own rule right now; I want to bow before myself in worship as I yield to my own will; I want to indulge myself because I know better than God knows; I want to glory in my sinful pleasures and live for my glory alone."

This is the true outworking of covetousness, the ultimate meaning of idolatry, and the wicked howl of a wretched heart, which screeches in demonic and diabolical intonations, *Autonomy! Autonomy! Autonomy! I will attain ultimate fulfillment through my own devices—fully independent of God. I will make my own call on what is good and what is evil. I will ascend above the heights of the clouds, and I will be like the Most High.*

Trendsetters Wanted

So there you have it—discontent, disbelief, and deification—the satanic playbook in all its insidious glory. This is the trap, the one that Beelzebub set for our forerunners, the one he has since set for every one of their descendants, and the one we have watched him set before our very eyes. Yes, the one we've knowingly walked into repeatedly and will continue to walk into endlessly if we don't do something drastic to change the trend.

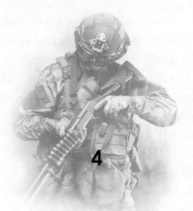

4

BLITZKRIEG

THE DEVIL'S PLAYBOOK FOR SEXUAL TEMPTATIONS

Discontent: Satanic Whispers

Here's how Satan's ancient and immutable blitzkrieg battle plan plays out when it comes to the area of sexual temptations. He begins by drawing our attention toward a particular sexual pleasure that God has expressly forbidden. Satan then magnifies that one thing to such an exaggerated degree that he blinds us to the countless other lawful pleasures that God has blessed us with. We suddenly find ourselves giving in to discontent, despising the blessings we do have and convincing ourselves that they avail us nothing until we can have that sinful, illicit pleasure.

And so, the devil's barrage of discombobulating lies begins:

> How unfair it is of God to give you a sex drive and not allow you to fulfill it. You're so young and far off from being married; how does God expect you to stay celibate for such a long time? You've been single for so many years, and who knows how long it will be before you'll marry? Why would God create you to be attracted to women and then not permit you to have satisfying sexual thoughts

about them in your mind or to enjoy the exhilarating thrill that comes from seeing them naked in photos or videos? Why would God allow your body to build such intense sexual tension and then not allow you to release it through masturbation? Why would God give you a wife, allow you to still feel attraction for other women, and then tell you that you can't have sex with them too? Yes, you have a wife, but in light of her having such a low sex drive, why are you still forbidden to find sexual release through other means? Is it fair that God gave you a wife but then took her away through death and now tells you that you can't have sex again unless you remarry?

You feel your defenses beginning to weaken as you slowly become consumed by the one thing that you can't have, and you start to despise every blessing that you do possess. Discontent starts to surge through you as you slowly become suspicious of God's goodness and believe that He must be unfair and uncaring toward you.

Disbelief: Irrational Rationalizations

As you try to regain your composure, you remind yourself that God has actually abundantly blessed you with more joys and pleasures than you can count. You also begin weighing the fact that your gracious Creator made it clear to you that sexual immorality is a unique sin against your own body and that there are radically severe consequences for it.

Your soul's greatest enemy can't contain himself any longer. He's a pathological liar of the highest order, and even though his first volley is usually laced with misleading elements, his preferred method of attack is unbridled and outright deceit. And so, he takes aim and fires away:

Come on, you know that God isn't going to do anything just because you go with what's natural. After all, God gave you a desire for sexual intimacy with a woman, and it's completely normal for you to get some release and satisfaction. You won't be harming your mind or your body; you'll actually be helping them reach a much-needed state of calm and relaxation, which is very good for you. You'll be doing the same for your partner, and this will draw you even closer to each other and strengthen your relational bonds. There won't be any negative consequences for this— only good ones.

At this point, your gaze has been fixed like a heat-seeking missile on the sexual temptation that tantalizingly dangles before your eyes. Reason has begun to give way to madness. *Wow! Is it really fair of God to tell me that I can't fulfill this natural desire that He Himself has given me? Why would He be trying to keep this from me? Are there really going to be negative consequences if I engage in something that feels so right and that brings such wonderful pleasure? I've seen plenty of people engage in various sexual activities for years, and nothing has happened to them. I'm sure I'll be fine.*

Deification: The God Delusion

With your defense walls completely decimated and your will to fight smashed to smithereens, Satan capitalizes on the enervated state of your soul, and he mercilessly drops "Tsar Bomba" on you with demonic glee. He diabolically lures your mind to think thoughts like these: *I'm sick and tired of being so sexually bound up. I feel like a worthless slave with no freedom. I long to finally be free to experience the thrill of sexual pleasure. I want to be able to do what I desire for once. This time, I'm doing it my way!*

And with that, you sink your teeth into the forbidden, command your phone to play your favorite exhilarating song, launch yourself toward the heights of the clouds, and seek to be like the Most High. But just before you clear the trees, your pathetic, homemade jet pack starts to sputter and run out of fuel, and you spiral toward the ground like a fat goose picked off in midair by a shotgun blast.

Dropping Like Dominoes

Having been duped into discontent, you yield to lustful covetousness. In this disenchanted state, you do the unthinkable and give in to disbelief about what God has said regarding the destructive consequences of sexual sin. After you're stunned by these two massive body blows, your discontent and disbelief give way to deification. Here, you essentially fashion yourself into your own god and then worshipfully sacrifice on the altar of your insolent rebellion and self-will the virtues of holiness, purity, integrity, humility, dependence, faithfulness, loyalty, and total surrender to the God who lavished you with unimaginable and undeserved blessings.

You would think that such a process takes hours or days, perhaps even weeks or months, to play itself out. And while in some cases it may, you can find yourself in most circumstances flying from step one to step three in a matter of moments.

Tragically, this self-sabotage traces its genesis back to Genesis. I can't say it better than Owen Strachan and Gavin Peacock did in their insightful book *What Does the Bible Teach about Lust?*: "The reason our vision of sex goes awry is because we followed the words of a snake over our Sovereign. It's true. Genesis 3 gives us the real historical narrative of our collective human breakdown. Our first father and mother trusted Satan over God, and believed his word over the Lord's."[1]

1   Gavin Peacock and Owen Strachan, *What Does the Bible Teach about Lust?: A Short Book on Desire* (Fearn, Ross-shire, UK: Christian Focus, 2020), 41.

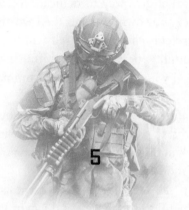

5

COUNTERATTACK

HOW TO BEAT THE DEVIL AT HIS OWN GAME

The Pouncing Prowler

So now what? Knowing the Enemy's battle plan and tactics will do us no good if we don't learn how to avoid his traps, fend him off, and go on the counterattack. We must follow Paul's strong appeal in 2 Corinthians 2:11 and not allow the Enemy to take advantage of us. And we do this by not being ignorant of his schemes. The wise Christian is ever mindful of the fact that Satan is constantly prowling around "like a roaring lion, seeking whom he may devour" (1 Peter 5:8). The operative word is *whom*. It should be every Christian man's intentional and burning passion to never qualify as a *whom*.

Before Peter identified Satan as a beast on the hunt, he gave us a fitting exhortation that helps protect us against our devouring adversary. He told us to be "sober" and "vigilant" (v. 8). *Barnes' Notes on the New Testament* sheds special light on the word *vigilant*. "This word… is everywhere else in the New Testament rendered 'watch,'" comparing it to references to Matthew 24:42–43; 25:13; 26:38; and 26:40–41 before stating, "It means that we should exercise careful circumspection, as one does when he is in danger."[1] Nothing is more conducive to stirring up watchfulness, careful circumspection, and a realization of the danger that Satan presents than understanding that he is a prowling lion who seeks to devour us.

Perhaps more than at any other time in world history, sobriety and vigilance are in dangerously short supply. The current generation has been lulled into an inebriated stupor by the intoxicating allurements of entertainment, materialism, and hedonism. And the resulting by-product is a careless, negligent, and lazy approach to the care of the soul.

Rise of the Resistance

After Peter clearly outlined Satan's destructive intentions toward the believer, he advised us how to combat him. He said, "Resist him, steadfast in the faith" (1 Peter 5:9). This coincides with what James 4:7 tells us: "Resist the devil and he will flee from you." And Paul, in Ephesians 6:16, said to take "the shield of faith with which you will be able to quench all the fiery darts of the wicked one."

When we think of resistance, our mind typically conjures up images of people fighting against an oppressive or encroaching enemy. We exert pressure and energy to fend against a harmful and destructive force. We fight off the unwanted. We battle the loathsome. We repel the tyrannical. Satan, however, has managed to become everyone's most beloved and cherished villain—a "frenemy" of sorts or a peculiarly avuncular fellow who brings us candy whenever he comes to visit but whom we know is simultaneously out to harm us. He's someone we're definitely wary of but on whom we've also become somewhat dependent. Kind of like a drug dealer who we know is contributing to our destruction but who is always faithful to deliver the addictive fix we desire.

Under what circumstances is it ever acceptable to consort with an enemy? When does that ever end well? And how contradictory is camaraderie to the very nature of animosity? Would a lioness ever welcome a hyena to watch over her cubs? Would a mouse cuddle up to a viper? Would a hen lay her eggs in a fox's den? Unthinkable. And yet, many Christians get much cozier with Satan than that.

---

1   Albert Barnes, *Barnes' Notes on the New Testament* (Grand Rapids, MI: Kregel Publications, 1962), 1435.

How, then, do we resist Satan firm in our faith, and how do we quench his fiery darts with the shield of faith? In keeping with the authoritative definition of *faith* found in God's Word, "Faith is the substance of things hoped for, the evidence of things not seen" (Hebrews 11:1), faith is best evidenced by actions that correspond to trust in what God has revealed is true before the outcome is realized. God tells us that it is right to flee youthful lusts, and He makes it clear that sexual immorality results in severe consequences because it's a distinct sin that we commit against our own body. A person demonstrating true faith responds with actions that reflect a sincere belief in what God has said. And they do this despite what they may think or feel.

A Workhorse Named Faith

Christians rarely get tripped up more than they do when it comes to walking in faith. We often have a hard time understanding what walking in faith really means. And yet, grasping the simplicity of how to do it can be one of the most freeing elements imaginable and one that will serve us as an extremely powerful and effective weapon in resisting Satan.

Generally speaking, just about everything God calls us to do requires faith on our part. Our problem is that we often equate genuine faith with supportive thoughts and cooperative emotions. While those elements can exist when we exercise our faith, they are not actual components of faith. Faith is not some mystical, esoteric, ambiguous, and elusive abstraction. It's a concrete reality that we can be certain we possess, and when we've legitimately exercised it, we undoubtedly know that we have.

While the book of Hebrews gives us perspective on what faith actually is, James delivers eye-opening truth that contains power that is revolutionary and paradigm shifting: "Faith by itself, if it does not have works, is dead. But someone will say, 'You have faith, and I have works.' Show me your faith without your works, and I will show you my faith by my works" (2:17–18). James was making it emphatically clear to us that there is a way through which we can clearly and undeniably show that we have faith. He told us that we do this by our works—by what we do in connection with what we claim to believe.

Of course, it's possible for religious hypocrites to go through the motions of fulfilling righteous deeds and yet have a heart that is not legitimately inclined to honor God. But I'm talking about the genuine believer who sincerely loves God and who truly desires to glorify Him but who is simultaneously battling undesired thoughts and emotions that conflict with what they truly believe. How does this type of person demonstrate their faith by their works when their faith is challenged?

God's Word explicitly teaches us that prayer is important. In our spirit, we believe that, but like Jesus said in the garden of Gethsemane to the disciples who kept falling asleep when He asked them to watch and pray, "The spirit indeed is willing, but the flesh is weak" (Matthew 26:41). So while we believe that prayer is important, all sorts of contrary thoughts and emotions will bombard our hearts and minds, telling us that it's not important to us. This is when we often surmise that we are defeated and that we must not truly believe prayer is important. And from here everything can quickly go south.

We mistakenly conclude that because we don't think or feel that we have faith, we can't do what's right, and at this point, we begin to stray. However, this is the exact juncture where we can show our faith by our works. We prove that we believe prayer is important by willing ourselves into prayer despite what we may feel or think. We don't have to wonder if we believe; we can know we do by the genuine works we execute in alignment with the things we genuinely believe.

We can say the same for reading and studying the Bible, giving generously toward God's work, acting with forgiveness toward those who have wronged us, proclaiming the gospel, sacrificing our time to serve others, and the list could go on and on.

Flood Control

Generally speaking, doing what God teaches is how we resist the devil firm in our faith; this is how we quench his fiery darts with the shield of faith. So how do we specifically do this when it comes to the area of sexual temptations?

When Satan comes rushing in like a flood with a barrage of destructive lies, we must counter him by proclaiming God's truth to ourselves and then willing ourselves into producing faith-filled works that are consistent with the biblical truths we believe—no matter what contrary thoughts or emotions we might be having at that moment. We do this by activating the self-control we can access through the fruit of the Spirit.

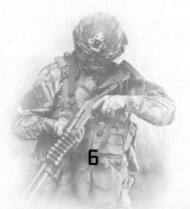

6

HOW TO DECIMATE DISCONTENT

Beyond Your Wildest Dreams

If ever there were a darling sin that the majority of God's people universally coddle, it would unquestionably be the sin of discontent. It's equally as deceptive as it is destructive. Because it's so prevalent among Christians, it's easy for believers to become desensitized to how serious, harmful, and dishonoring to God discontent really is.

In his powerfully convicting book *The Art of Divine Contentment*, Thomas Watson struck more than a few chords when he revealed the true nature and corrosive effects of discontent: "Discontent is a fretting humour, which dries the brains, wastes the spirits, corrodes and eats out the comfort of life; discontent makes a man that he doth not enjoy what he doth possess. A drop or two of vinegar will sour a whole glass of wine. Let a man have the affluence and confluence of worldly comforts, a drop or two of discontent will embitter and poison all."[1]

He then targeted discontent's rotten fruit: "Murmuring is no better than mutiny in the heart; it is a rising up against God. When the sea is rough and unquiet, it casts forth nothing but foam: when the heart is discontented, it casts forth the foam of anger, impatience, and sometimes

---

1   Thomas Watson, *The Art of Divine Contentment: An Exposition of Philippians 4:11* (Glasgow, UK: Free Presbyterian Publications, 1855), 19, https://grace-ebooks.com.

FIGHT LIKE A MAN

little better than blasphemy. Murmuring is nothing else but the scum which boils off from a discontented heart."[2]

When Satan attempts to lure you toward discontent by highlighting the fact that God has restricted you from partaking of the forbidden fruit of sexual sin, you must immediately raise up your shield of faith and quench his fiery darts. You do that by choosing to believe that God has given you more than you could have ever dreamed of, both physically and spiritually. Despite your current frustrations with being denied the freedom to indulge in unlawful sexual desires, you count your blessings and acknowledge the plethora of other pleasures God has allowed you to enjoy. While all our circumstances are different and some of us may have some extremely painful and challenging ones, surely we can all find plenty of things in our lives to be grateful for. Things such as enriching friendships; a loving family; a comfortable home; plenty of clothing; a consistent job; the ability to hear beautiful music, to see God's breathtaking creation, to taste delicious and satisfying food; the capacity to think and reason and communicate; the pleasure of reading, writing, and resting; the enjoyment of art, poetry, and fashion; and so much more.

It Gets Even Better

On top of the physical blessings, we possess far more important spiritual ones. Ephesians 1:3 tells us that we've been blessed "with every spiritual blessing in the heavenly places." And from there, Paul went on to enumerate and elaborate on the indescribable wealth we possess in Christ: our election, our predestination, our adoption, our redemption, our forgiveness, our inheritance, our sealing in the Holy Spirit. And as if that weren't enough, Scripture calls Jesus our Good Shepherd. Unlike the masses in Mark 6 and Matthew 9, whom He looked upon with compassion—seeing them as weary and scattered, like sheep having no shepherd—Jesus sees us as the sheep of His pasture, and He lavishes us with His provision, His guidance, and His protection.

But it doesn't stop there. Jesus continues to bless us with the indescribable treasure that is the body of Christ. He guards us and guides us by brightly shining the light of His immutable Word. He comforts and enlightens us through the presence of His Holy Spirit. And He grants us

2   Watson, *The Art of Divine Contentment*, 14.

the grace of being heirs of His eternal, heavenly kingdom, promising that we will one day rule and reign with Him over the new earth.

Not as Bad as You Thought

Now take all those unspeakable and undeserved blessings and consider them against the backdrop of our dark and depraved hearts, our wickedly blasphemous deeds, and our wretched rebellion against the gracious God who has graced us with such unfathomable goodness. Then add to that the consideration of what we truly deserve because of our sinfulness compared to the light circumstances that we may be experiencing. Ephesians 2 tells us that we were at one time children of wrath. Our offenses against a holy God have earned us the eternal judgment of what the Bible calls the "lake of fire" (Revelation 20:11–15; 21:8). In fact, that is where we literally should be right now, but we're not. This knowledge will help transform our thinking and give us the proper perspective as we face our challenging and painful hardships.

Smaller Than You Remember

With this sort of mindset and attitude, our heart becomes fortified against Satan's temptation toward discontent. As we meditate on all the pleasures and blessings with which God has enriched our lives, our outlook begins to change. It's further transformed when we consider the fact that we actually deserve the lake of fire in place of our present circumstances. Deep gratitude fills our heart, and thanksgiving flows from our lips as we realize that instead of struggling with mere disappointment because we cannot indulge our self-willed and unlawful sexual passions, we should be presently engulfed in eternal flames. Suddenly, we see the tree bearing the forbidden fruit, which seemed to be the size of the whole planet, for the microscopic restriction that it is when compared to all the amazing gifts God has showered us with. And we become keenly conscious of the fact that the command to abstain is a rich display of God's protective love over us. We find ourselves less and less consumed with that one thing that we can't have. And instead of persisting in the sin of Haman, who lamented that the plethora of amazing things that he possessed tragically availed him nothing, our abundant blessings regain their proper place in our hearts, benefiting us greatly in our battle against discontent and sexual sin.

And this should be no wonder to us. Scripture makes it abundantly clear that doing things God's way has its perks: "Godliness with contentment is great gain" (1 Timothy 6:6). I'll close this chapter with these discontent-decimating words from Heath Lambert:

> Gratitude is the attitude of a heart that is thankful for anything and everything the Lord gives. You are grateful when you are glad for and content with what you have. Thankfulness is the opposite of lust because the thankful heart has stopped prowling around for everything it doesn't have and is overwhelmed with appreciation for all the good things it already possesses. The logic of lust requires you to be discontent with what you have and pay attention to all the things you don't have. The logic of thankfulness requires you to focus on what you have already received and to be overcome with thanks. Gratitude is the opposite of greed.[3]

3   Heath Lambert, *Finally Free: Fighting for Purity with the Power of Grace* (Grand Rapids, MI: Zondervan, 2013), 126.

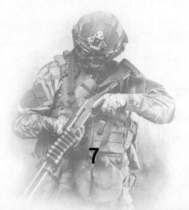

7

HOW TO DEFEAT DISBELIEF

A Very Sinful Sin

Having neutralized Satan's attempt to lure us into discontent and entice us to question God's kindness and care for us, we now need to continue our proactive campaign of intentional resistance as the devil seeks to flood our minds with disbelief over God's promised consequences for our sexual sin.

One of modern Christianity's most popular mantras is "Sin is sin." What's implied by this is that all sin is equal. While it's true that all sin is equal in the sense that all sin is equally a violation of God's holy standards, all sin is not equal in terms of its impact, its egregiousness, and its consequences. For example, if I lie to you about having other plans when you ask me to help you move to a new house, I've undoubtedly committed a sin. However, its impact, egregiousness, and consequences would not be the same as if I had murdered your entire family.

When speaking of sexual sin, Paul the Apostle said this in 1 Corinthians 6:18: "Flee sexual immorality. Every sin that a man does is outside the body, but he who commits sexual immorality sins against his own body." Paul minced no words here when he juxtaposed sexual sin with what he called the sins that man commits "outside the body," thus highlighting sexual sin as distinctly and exceedingly sinful. God's Word is also perfectly clear when it says that "fornicators and adulterers God will judge" (Hebrews 13:4) and that the "sexually immoral…shall have their part in the lake which burns with fire and brimstone" (Revelation 21:8).

Cause and Effect

Sexual sin has massive repercussions. It's not to be trifled with. There is no escape from the dire warning we're given in Galatians 6:7–8: "Do not be deceived, God is not mocked; for whatever a man sows, that he will also reap. For he who sows to his flesh will of the flesh reap corruption, but he who sows to the Spirit will of the Spirit reap everlasting life."

Sowing to the flesh by indulging in sexual sin through the gateway of lust will indeed lead to massive corruption. As we discover in *Passions of the Heart*, "This is because lust robs you of a passion for godliness and righteousness; it replaces holy lust with unholy lust. It promotes a love for self above a love for God and others. It assaults your conscience, weakening your sense of guilt and culpability, and sears it with the hot iron of indifference. It defiles your character and opens the floodgates of doubt, jealousy, and distrust."[1]

As he did with Eve, Satan will seek to convince you that God didn't really mean what He said regarding the severity of sexual sin and its destructive consequences. He wants you to buy into the audaciously preposterous lie that the one who is the very definition of perfection itself has somehow suddenly decided to deviate from His immutable nature.

Few words about sexual immorality are as sobering as the ones that the Holy Spirit penned through the apostle Paul in the book of Ephesians: "This you know, that no fornicator, unclean person, nor covetous man, who is an idolater, has any inheritance in the kingdom of Christ and God. Let no one deceive you with empty words, for because of these things the wrath of God comes upon the sons of disobedience. Therefore do not be partakers with them" (5:5–7).

The warning here is quite clear. First, we see that those who are engaged in sexual immorality will not inherit the kingdom of God. Next, God's Word reveals to us that deceptive words will accost us and will seek

---

1   John D. Street, *Passions of the Heart: Biblical Counsel for Stubborn Sexual Sins* (Phillipsburg, NJ: P&R Publishing, 2019), 257–58.

to dupe us into believing that God will not really bar from His kingdom those who live in sexual sin. Then, Paul's letter assures us that, in reality, God will pour out His wrath on those who live sinfully rebellious lives. And finally, Scripture warns us not to be partakers with them. In other words, Paul exhorted us not to do the things that they do.

He Can See Right through You

At this point, you might be thinking, *But I thought that a believer's salvation is eternally secured by the finished work of Christ.* You're absolutely right. If you have been spiritually quickened and regenerated by the Spirit of God, then it holds indisputably true that He has sealed you and has guaranteed your eternal inheritance (Ephesians 1:13–14). However, if someone professes faith in Christ yet continues to engage in sexual immorality, he would be wise to do as Scripture says and examine himself to see if he's truly in the faith (2 Corinthians 13:5) and to make his "call and election sure" (2 Peter 1:10).

It seems to almost shock the modern man when he hears that it's possible for someone to profess to be a Christian and not really be one. But God's Word makes it clear that this can most definitely be the case. Titus 1:16 says, "They profess to know God, but in works they deny Him." As 1 John 1:5–6 declares, "This is the message which we have heard from Him and declare to you, that God is light and in Him is no darkness at all. If we say that we have fellowship with Him, and walk in darkness, we lie and do not practice the truth." And the same epistle goes on to say, "Now by this we know that we know Him, if we keep His commandments. He who says, 'I know Him,' and does not keep His commandments, is a liar, and the truth is not in him" (2:3–4).

Jesus made it very clear in Matthew 7 that many will call Him "Lord, Lord" (v. 21) on the day of judgment but that He will say to them, "I never knew you," because they "practice lawlessness" (v. 23). This is an extremely sobering thought. Actually, it's almost traumatizing. The last thing any of us wants to believe is that we might not be saved. But we should be willing to go through the pain of considering that now rather than the inexplicable horror of hearing those words from Christ on that great and terrible day.

If Satan has been victorious over you in an area as crucial as disbelief, then resisting him on the other two fronts we've examined will be moot. In fact, you won't even have the wherewithal to resist him. So dive deep into this urgent exploration and don't handle yourself with kid gloves. There are many real-life accounts of even pastors who eventually discovered that they weren't genuinely saved.

How to Make a Parachute Feel Softer Than a Pillow

The best place to start exploring the genuineness of your salvation is by examining your initial motives for coming to Christ in the first place. Unfortunately, because of how a multitude of modern preachers have twisted the gospel, many have the impression that Jesus is a means to their best life now, complete with health, wealth, and a carefree existence full of ultra-happiness. When this is our motive for pursuing Christ, then we are not really pursuing Christ. The object of pursuit becomes a celestial genie who will serve us hand and foot, standing ready to fulfill our every selfish whim. This is not the Christ of Scripture, and this is not the motive that will lead to genuine conversion. This is a false Christ and a carnal, man-centered pseudo-gospel.

As Ray Comfort so aptly described in his famous sermon "Hell's Best Kept Secret," many preachers tell people that if they put Jesus on like a parachute in an airplane, He'll improve their flight, making them more comfortable and helping them enjoy their journey. But when they suddenly discover that sitting in their airplane seat with a parachute on their back is actually extremely uncomfortable, they become embittered toward the parachute and toward those who advised them to put it on. Thus, they proceed to quickly throw it off. However, if they had been told that the airplane was malfunctioning and that they should put the parachute on because, within moments, they will have to take a treacherous jump thousands of feet into the air, then the entire situation would have suddenly transformed. They would hardly notice the discomfort of the parachute on their back as they sat in their seat, and the more difficult the flight became, the tighter they would cling to the parachute. And why is this? It's because they put the parachute on for the right reason. They put it on not to improve their flight but to be saved during the jump that is to come.[2]

Grass, Snow, Sheep, and Hitler

So why did you put on the Lord Jesus Christ? Was it for life-enhancement purposes, or was it because you saw yourself as a sinner in desperate need of the Savior? You may say, *Sure that was somewhere in the mix. I mean, everyone sins, but I've actually always been a pretty good person.* Our problem as people is that we often compare ourselves to others, and on that basis, we minimize the seriousness of our sinfulness against an infinitely holy God. The man who smokes weed thinks he's a pretty good guy when he compares himself to the person slamming heroin. The heroin addict will console himself by thinking that at least he's never hurt anyone like the rapist has. The rapist, as horrified as he should be by his heinous crimes, will point to the murderer and say, "At least I've never taken anyone's life." Even the murderer will conclude that he's a pretty good guy when he points to someone like Hitler, who murdered millions. As it has been said, a white sheep grazing in a pasture looks quite white against the backdrop of the green grass. But if you were to look at that same sheep in the same pasture after a snowstorm, it wouldn't look so white anymore with that pure-white, snowy background.

In light of that and in order for us to examine the true state of our soul before a God of impeccable righteousness, we have to look at His moral law as the standard of measure. The Ten Commandments work like a mirror: they reflect back to us who we really are. With that in mind, let me hold up the mirror and allow it to help you discover what's true about your reflection.

If you were to take a guess, how many lies would you estimate you've told over the course of your lifetime? For some reason, we like to assign sizes and colors to lies—"little" and "white" seem to be top favorites. But the Bible makes it clear that liars will not inherit the kingdom of God. If you've ever stolen something, regardless of its value or how long ago you stole it, you'd be guilty of being a thief. Have you ever used God's name in vain? Think about it; we don't do this with the names of some of history's most atrocious villains—like Stalin or Mussolini—but we do it

2   Ray Comfort, "Hell's Best Kept Secret," Living Waters, July 27, 2019, https://livingwaters.com.

with the name of the God who gave us life and everything that we enjoy in it. The Bible calls this blasphemy, and it assures us that God will not hold him guiltless who takes His name in vain. Jesus equated lust with adultery, and the Bible likens unjust anger and hatred to murder.

The worst news of all is that Scripture tells us that if we've sinned in one point of God's law, we're guilty of breaking the whole thing. And the heinous nature of sin is magnified all the more when we realize that we've repeatedly sinned against a God who has magnanimously lavished us with more loving-kindness than we could ever account for. When we couple that with the fact that the Lord is infinitely holy and perfectly just, we can see why hell is an appropriate penalty for those who have willfully violated the law of such a God—those who are, in reality, liars, thieves, blasphemers, adulterers, and murderers.

The Hero Dying for the Villain?

Now here is where God's love leaves us speechless. Despite our unspeakable wickedness, rebellion, and depravity—which were manifested by a life of blasphemous contempt and outright hatred toward the one who lavishes us with innumerable graces—God chose to do the unthinkable for His wretched foes. He left the heights of heaven, took upon Himself the form of a man, subjected Himself to the rejection and torment inflicted by His own creation, and ultimately allowed Himself to be brutally murdered not only *by* His enemies but also *for* them.

This is how God simultaneously demonstrated justice and mercy, judgment and grace. He demonstrated justice and judgment by pouring out His wrath on account of the violation of His holy law. He demonstrated mercy and grace by pouring that wrath out on His own Son, who willingly took the place of sinners, lived the perfect life they could never live, and became their substitute on the cross. This means that all those who repent of their sins and believe that Christ died and rose again as God's propitiation—in other words, as the one who turned away God's wrath through His shed blood for violators of His righteous standard—will be forgiven of every sin they've ever committed, will receive the perfect righteousness of Christ as a free gift, and will inherit everlasting life.

My hope is that if you recognize that you did not originally come to Christ with the right motives, you'll do so now. While even freedom from an addiction to pornography should not be your motive for surrendering your life to Christ, being genuinely born again and having the power of God's Spirit dwelling in you are the most effective route to unshackling yourself from Satan's enslaving grip.

The Mirror Never Lies

I would imagine that, at this point, you've probably identified one of three things to be true about yourself in connection with Satan's foundational tactic of luring people toward unbelief in the gospel. First, perhaps you acknowledged that you have never identified as a Christian, have never believed the claims of Christianity, and still don't. Second, maybe you recognized that you truly did believe with the right motives at the time of your profession of faith in Christ, and you were a true Christian from that point. And third, it could be that you just realized that you were never genuinely saved but have now come to true repentance toward God and a sincere faith in Jesus Christ.

If you can relate to the first description, please don't stop reading this book. I'm so grateful you picked it up, and I hope that by the time you get to the end of it, God will have drawn you to a firm belief in the gospel. However, if you find yourself aligning with what I outlined in the second or third descriptions, then let me now explain to you how you can proactively fight against Satan's attempts to lure you into disbelief about what God has said about the consequences of sexual sin.

He's Not Bluffing

She was frazzled, frustrated, and on the brink of blowing her top. Disneyland is brutal enough with its endless lines, massive shoulder-to-shoulder crowds, and $20,000 bags of cotton candy. (I'm slightly exaggerating about the endless lines.) But add one-hundred-degree, sweltering heat to that, and you end up with a recipe for disaster. Her three little ones would not stop testing her patience. You saw them running away from her near the Dumbo ride, pulling on Goofy's tail in Mickey's Toontown, and trying to climb the side of the Matterhorn. Each time, she threatened to take them home if they didn't stop what they were doing by the count of three, and each time, they continued disobeying when she reached three (even after the painfully protracted "Two and a haaaaaaaaalf"), and each time, she failed to make good on the promised consequences.

This illustration is not far off from many people's outlook on the nature of God's consistency when dispensing consequences for sins. They imagine Him to be "the God of the empty threat." He huffs and puffs to scare us into submission, and when we don't submit, well, He usually does nothing about it. Simply stated, we end up deceiving ourselves into believing that we can somehow mock God.

Scripture, however (as I've already mentioned), makes it extremely clear (in Galatians 6:7–8) that we shouldn't be "deceived" into thinking that we can mock God and not end up reaping what we sow. The Bible specifically warns us not to be deceived because this false concept of God not following through on dispensing consequences for sin is obviously extremely deceptive. So our first countermeasure against Satan is to remind ourselves that we can't pull a fast one on God.

In much the same way that we can't jump off a fifty-story building and mock the law of gravity by not violently colliding with the pavement, so it is that we can't sin sexually without reaping the consequences of corruption in our lives. We need to meditate on the biblical accounts that clearly highlight the corruption of those who sowed to the flesh and of God's faithful discipline toward His children who have rebelled against Him—from Adam and Eve to Moses, to Jonah, to David, to Sampson, to Ananias and Sapphira. And this is just a very small sampling.

It would do us well to remember the indisputable words found in Scripture:

> Can a man take fire to his bosom,
> and his clothes not be burned?
> Can one walk on hot coals,
> and his feet not be seared? (Proverbs 6:27–28)

We Aim to Please

Along with being gripped by the fact that our immorality will incur God's discipline in a temporal sense, another helpful strategy to defeat sexual sin is to grasp the reality that our sexual sins will have eternal consequences by way of causing us to forfeit certain heavenly rewards. We should be radically sobered by the realization that there is coming a day when we will stand before God to give an account for how we conducted ourselves on this earth. Paul's words should serve us all as a jolting wake-up call: "We must all appear before the judgment seat of Christ, that each one may receive the things done in the body, according to what he has done, whether good or bad" (2 Corinthians 5:10).

While it's a relief to know that this is not the great white throne judgment of Revelation 20—where God will dispense condemnation to unrepentant unbelievers—it will nonetheless be a serious day of reckoning for the Christian. This is what Scripture calls the judgment seat of Christ, and Scripture makes it clear that we will forfeit our rewards based on our disobedience and sin (1 Corinthians 3:11–15). We'll explore this in depth later in the book.

But far beyond the loss of reward, we should be shaken to our core by the thought of looking into the eyes of the Redeemer, who paid such a high price to ransom our souls. In fact, Jesus paid the highest price ever paid for anything ever purchased in the history of the universe. Envision yourself giving an account before such a loving Savior for perverse sexual sins that you committed in His presence—in the very shadow of His cross. Imagine having loudly declared, through your actions, that His sacrifice didn't really mean anything to you.

Now remember, if you've been genuinely born again, as severe as your sexual sins may have been, God will by no means pour out any condemnation on you. He paid for those sins on the cross by receiving condemnation in your place—the very condemnation you deserved. And that's why God's Word clearly tells us, "There is therefore now no condemnation to those who are in Christ Jesus" (Romans 8:1).

However, this very fact should overwhelm you with deep gratitude and passionately compel you to never want to displease such a benevolent Savior. Is this not the sentiment with which Paul preceded his warning about the judgment seat of Christ? "We make it our aim, whether present or absent, to be well pleasing to Him" (2 Corinthians 5:9).

"I'm Glad I Did"

If you've ever watched the hidden camera social experiment program *What Would You Do?*, you've tasted what regret can look like. The program format usually involves actors playing out a variety of scenarios in a setting like a store or restaurant. For example, one person might pretend to bully another or to make racist comments toward people or to be abusive toward their spouse or child or to steal something from someone else. The hidden cameras then capture the reactions of unsuspecting people who witness the bad behavior. Inevitably, once things have played out long enough, the host, John Quiñones, and his camera crew will come out and interview the bystanders.

More often than not, those who witnessed these terrible offenses but chose to cower and do nothing will say to the interviewer, "I wish I would have." But those who defended the victims or spoke up for the cause of justice will typically look into the camera and say, "I'm glad I did."

Likewise, you can be one of two types of people as you stand before the judgment seat of Christ after having faced the temptation of sexual immorality. You can either be the "I wish I would have" type of person or the "I'm glad I did" type of person. Which will you choose to be?

Don't give in to Satan's temptation toward disbelief when it comes to the regretful consequences that God has promised will result when we indulge in sexual immorality. And if you're thinking to yourself, *But I've already committed sexual sins—even as a Christian*, then recognize that there is hope for you in the grace and mercy of God. Don't be one who will have to say on that day, "I wish I would have repented and fully cut off my intermittent lapses into sexual sin." Be the kind of person who will say, "I'm glad I did."

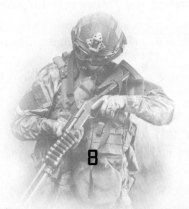

8

HOW TO DESTROY DEIFICATION

Raising the Iron Dome

At this point in resisting Satan "steadfast in the faith" (1 Peter 5:9), we've learned how to dodge his bullet of discontent and avoid his heat-seeking missile of disbelief. More than that, we've become equipped to go on the offensive and gain victory over his relentless onslaughts in these two areas of attack. Now it's time to explore how to go toe to toe with him and defeat him in the face of his most lethal attack of all—the nuclear bomb of deification.

The Very Extraordinary and Legendary Larry

It was a typical open-air outreach at our regular preaching spot at the Third Street Promenade in Santa Monica. Ray Comfort was preaching the Word of God when a very interesting character began to heckle him. Now contrary to what many might expect, Ray actually prays that God will bring him hecklers. Their passion and intensity usually enlarge the crowd, and more people end up hearing the gospel. If hecklers received a grade, this guy would have definitely gotten an A+ in his honors heckling class.

He began speaking with a very deep, booming voice, and in impressive King James English, he proclaimed himself to be God. He got on a roll, describing the greatness of his deity in lofty and self-aggrandizing terms.

After letting him drone on for a bit, Ray finally yelled out, "What's your name?"

Without skipping a beat, our friend immediately transitioned from his deep-voiced, King James English, self-deifying tirade to a rather unimpressive and relatively wimpy voice and said, "Larry."

Wow! We got to meet the Legendary Lord Larry? It was hard to hold back the laughter, and Ray and I have had many good laughs over that for years. What a good illustration this is of how silly man looks and sounds when he tries to usurp the throne of God Almighty.

As we've already seen, the temptation that Satan most often delights to use against us is the sin that brought about his own downfall—the wicked pride that seeks to dethrone God and take His place. How irrationally senseless is that? One would think that it's so utterly unbelievable that no one would be foolish enough to even imagine that taking the place of God is a real possibility. But it's important to bear in mind that Satan often veils his temptations with the illusion of reasonableness. He doesn't come out and directly lure you into literally saying, "I want to be like God and sit on His throne." He disguises the sin he wants you to commit as a necessary pursuit that you're entitled to. It's your right, and God is unjust to keep you from it.

Ice Bucket Challenge—with Extra Ice

A number of years ago, a very popular trend took the social media world by storm. It was called the Ice Bucket Challenge. Its purpose was to promote awareness of amyotrophic lateral sclerosis (ALS) and raise funds for research toward a cure. During the campaign's peak, you could hardly go on any social media platform without seeing someone allowing a friend to dump a bucket of ice water over their head and then challenging a few other people by name to allow someone to do the same thing to them. Even notable celebrities got in on the action. As stoic as some people tried to remain, inevitably their faces would involuntarily contort, their bodies would shiver, and their vocal cords would suddenly manifest a mind of their own, hitting frequencies that could almost shatter glass.

I think every man needs to get doused with some good, old-fashioned spiritual ice water. We need something outside us to shake us to our core and do something inside us, ultimately causing us to react in radical ways against the temptation to usurp the throne of God. We need something to severely jolt us and snatch us from the destructive pursuit of self-deification and autonomy, which is the by-product of indulging in sexual immorality.

Lightning and Fire

Proverbs makes it clear that "it is not good for a soul to be without knowledge" (19:2). Knowledge will be your greatest ally in the fight against Satan's lure toward deification. You must begin with the knowledge that the most destructive force in your existence is your reign over the affairs of your own life.

But before you look at yourself, it is wise to begin by examining how things turned out for others who insisted on supplanting God's reign over their lives. The best place to start is at the very beginning. Here you might think that I'm referring to the fall of Adam and Eve. While this is undoubtedly a monumentally infamous event that we will examine next, I think it would be good to go back even further and revisit what we lightly touched on earlier—the first sin ever committed in the history of the universe—the very sin that caused the fall of Satan, which, in turn, influenced the first human sin.

Isaiah 14 gives us keen insight into the repercussions of Satan's sin. While the passage directly deals with the king of Babylon, it seems clear that the diabolical entity behind the king is none other than Lucifer. This is evident, in part, by the fact that the passage mentions certain things that cannot pertain to that earthly king. We see that Lucifer fell from heaven and was cast down to the earth. Jesus said in Luke 10:18 that He "saw Satan fall like lightning from heaven." And Revelation 9:1 likens Satan to a star that fell from the sky to the earth. This seems to align with Satan's reply in the book of Job when God asked him where he came from: "From going to and fro on the earth, and from walking back and forth on it" (Job 1:7).

So Satan's first judgment was to be cast out of heaven, but his final judgment will be the eternal lake of fire (Revelation 20:10). And he won't be alone in this judgment, as he'll be joined by his demonic horde of fallen angels (2 Peter 2:4; Matthew 25:41). The demonic realm undoubtedly knew of this severe, pending judgment, as is evidenced by how Legion responded to Christ before He cast them into the swine: "Suddenly they cried out, saying, 'What have we to do with You, Jesus, You Son of God? Have You come here to torment us before the time?'" (Matthew 8:29).

The Bite Heard around the World

Turning now to the fall of man, aided by the devil's wiles after his expulsion from heaven, we see God uphold the same response to sin, a precedent that has never been broken—never! In Genesis, Satan said, "Eat and you will become like God"; God said, "Eat and you will die" (this meant physical and spiritual death—which also involves the consequence of hell for sinners who don't repent and trust Christ for salvation). Whose word was fulfilled?

This is the epitome of reaping and sowing. It's a perfect example of how one decision—one single foolish action executed in just a split second—can result in the most colossal and decimating of consequences imaginable.

The devastating judgment that Adam and Eve received from God because of their blatant defiance of His command should eliminate any ambiguity in our minds about God's perspective on sin. We tend to downplay the seriousness of sin in God's sight. We might be tempted to think that God wouldn't be too concerned with a little bit of lust, porn, or premarital sex. But the fact that the whole of creation was so severely and extensively cursed because a man and a woman ate a piece of forbidden fruit in a garden thousands of years ago reveals a deeper principle that goes beyond our actual acts of defiance.

From a Palace to a Pasture

Nebuchadnezzar was one of the greatest kings to ever strut across the stage of human history. Scripture makes it clear that although he was a pagan king, God Himself had commissioned his rule and even called Nebuchadnezzar His servant (Jeremiah 27:6). There came a day when Nebuchadnezzar was deeply troubled by a dream he had. After summoning Daniel to give him the interpretation, Nebuchadnezzar discovered that God was warning him about a severe judgment that was going to befall him because of his pride.

Here are the sobering words that Daniel spoke to him: "They shall drive you from men, your dwelling shall be with the beasts of the field, and they shall make you eat grass like oxen. They shall wet you with the dew of heaven, and seven times shall pass over you, till you know that the Most High rules in the kingdom of men, and gives it to whomever He chooses" (Daniel 4:25).

One might rightly conclude that this dire warning would have compelled Nebuchadnezzar to stay as far away as possible from anything that could bring about such a severe judgment. We might think this prophecy would rouse the same type of urgency toward repentance that we saw in the Ninevites when Jonah cried out, "Yet forty days, and Nineveh shall be overthrown!" (Jonah 3:4). Unfortunately, however, just as Christ warned Peter that before the rooster crowed, Peter would deny Him three times, and still Peter denied Him that very night—even after saying, "Even if I have to die with You, I will not deny You!" (Matthew 26:35)—so we see Nebuchadnezzar doing the same sort of thing: "All this came upon King Nebuchadnezzar. At the end of the twelve months he was walking about the royal palace of Babylon. The king spoke, saying, 'Is not this great Babylon, that I have built for a royal dwelling by my mighty power and for the honor of my majesty?'" (Daniel 4:28–30).

After this act of pride and self-deification, we're told the following: "That very hour the word was fulfilled concerning Nebuchadnezzar; he was driven from men and ate grass like oxen; his body was wet with the dew of heaven till his hair had grown like eagles' feathers and his nails like birds' claws" (v. 33).

Imagine that for a moment. The mighty king who subdued nations, conquered kingdoms, and ruled over vast portions of the planet was crawling around like an animal and eating grass. At the end of this tragic ordeal, after Nebuchadnezzar came to his senses and was restored to his kingdom, here's how he summed up the grand lesson he learned from the intense affliction he suffered at the hand of the God before whom he had dared to exalt himself: "Those who walk in pride He is able to put down" (v. 37).

Lord of the Worms

Our final example takes us to the New Testament era and gives us a glimpse into the tragic end of another king. While this ruler received no direct warning, he would have no doubt been familiar with the warnings connected to the biblical accounts we just explored. Herod Agrippa I was the fifth of six Herods who ruled over Israel. Herod the Great, Herod Archelaus, Herod Antipas, and Herod Philip preceded him. Finally, Herod Agrippa II succeeded him. Because of the Herod dynasty's close association with Rome, it's easy to assume that all the Herods were of Roman heritage. However, they were actually of Idumean and Arabian descent and had intermingled some elements from Judaism into their religious practices. Having ruled over the Jews for generations, they were also well-versed in the Jewish faith. For this reason, I highlight that Herod Agrippa I would have had intimate knowledge of the warnings given to the Old Testament figures we discussed previously. Nonetheless, the hypnotic lure of self-deification drew him to the brink of the abyss of self-destruction, and here's how he took the plunge:

> Herod had been very angry with the people of Tyre and Sidon; but they came to him with one accord, and having made Blastus the king's personal aide their friend, they asked for peace, because their country was supplied with food by the king's country.
>
> So on a set day Herod, arrayed in royal apparel, sat on his throne and gave an oration to them. And the people kept shouting, "The voice of a god and not of a man!" Then immediately an angel of the Lord struck him, because he did not give glory to God. And he was eaten by worms and died.
>
> But the word of God grew and multiplied.
> (Acts 12:20–24)

Frosty the No Man

Seeking to usurp the throne of almighty God is extremely dangerous business. His glory is not to be trifled with. When man is foolish enough to attempt to rob God of what belongs to Him, he soon learns that he would be more likely to succeed at building a snowman on the surface of the sun.

As we've seen from what happened with Satan, Adam and Eve, Nebuchadnezzar, and Herod Agrippa I (only a few out of many more examples available), when the Lord declares that there will be severe consequences for those who seek to play God, you can be sure that those consequences will unquestionably materialize.

Finally, do we really need a textbook lesson on how outrightly ignorant it is to deify ourselves and seek to rule over the affairs of our own lives by indulging in sexual immorality? How many times have we found ourselves shipwrecked on the shores of our idolatrous islands of rebellion in countless areas of our lives? Humans are microscopic beings who have no control over their own respiratory, cardiovascular, or digestive systems; who can't keep their hair from graying and falling out or their skin from wrinkling; and who sometimes can't even stop their own hiccups. Yet we would seriously seek to rule in the place of the infinite God of creation or think that we know better than He does about what's best for us. Really?

Battle Plan Recap

So it's here that we set our faces like flint, plant our feet like deep roots of iron, raise our shields high, and thrust relentlessly with our swords at an insidious enemy who would dare to whisper the slightest suggestion of mutiny against our sovereign Lord. We recall the fate of other would-be usurpers who suffered at the hands of their own arrogant folly and allow that to deter us from following in their footsteps.

This all culminates in our confession that only one rules supreme in the affairs of the universe and its inhabitants. We then remember that it's impossible for God to lie, and we arm ourselves with His unwavering Word about the devastating repercussions in our own lives if we dare seek to be like the Most High by attempting to establish our own standard of righteousness. Finally, we vigorously paddle against the riptide of a grumbling spirit by counting our blessings—refusing to act foolishly or to believe that these blessings avail us nothing because we can't carnally indulge in what God has lovingly declared is off-limits to us.

As we implement this battle plan against the Father of Lies and crucial victories begin to pile up, the winds of hope will fill our sails and drive us forward in our pursuit of sexual integrity. Discontent, disbelief, and deification will incrementally lose their grip on us. The joy of the Lord will be our strength as nearness to our precious Savior and uninterrupted communion with Him become more precious to us than the fading pleasures of sin.

But we have yet another enemy to conquer—the real enemy—the one who gives occasion to the devil and the world, who are merely the enemies of opportunity. Our flesh is lurking in the shadows, always waiting to pounce. We will now examine its schemes and formulate our plans for its crucifixion.

PART 2
THE FLESH

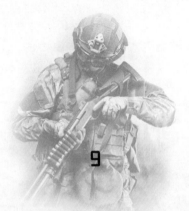

9

THE ENEMY WITHIN YOU

It's a Piece of Cake

I can't help but wonder how strange some of our Christianese lingo must sound to the ears of an unbeliever. Imagine having no Christian foundation whatsoever and then randomly hearing someone spit this rambling sentence at you: "I'm a blood-washed, regenerated, on-fire, sanctified saint who has girded my loins with truth and can faithfully wield the sword of the Spirit while holding up the shield of faith, bearing the fruit of agape, and persevering to the end because I've been sealed with the Holy Ghost."

It reminds me of when I immigrated to the United States from Lebanon at the age of four. I didn't speak a lick of English. I think the only things I knew how to say were "Hello" and "Give me chocolate!" Shortly after arriving at these glorious shores, my parents put me into a very dangerous, hostile, and deadly environment called kindergarten. It was strange to walk into the cafeteria expecting some hummus and baklava only to be greeted by something called a sloppy joe. Yeah, you guessed it: "Give me chocolate—*now!*"

Kindergarten definitely helped me build my vocabulary, but once I started to grasp conversational English, I encountered the wonderful world of abstract concepts—little elements that supersede basic, concrete paradigms. Idioms, in particular, were my least favorite abstractions (though I love them now). You know, those nifty sayings composed of words that have nothing to do with what someone actually means. Idioms like "over the moon" or "down in the mouth" or "piece of cake" or "break a leg." Imagine having no idea how English idioms work and then hearing your elementary school teacher tell you to "Get out there and break a leg" before going on stage to perform in your school play. Or your friend handing you a Rubik's Cube and saying, "Try it. It's a piece of cake." I'll let your imagination run wild with what the outcome might be if someone took those idioms literally (I'm glad I never did).

Similarly, as a new Christian, I was a bit befuddled when I first heard about this abstract concept called the flesh. Even as I wrote that just now, I found myself giggling when I remembered hearing it for the first time.

"Hey, don't walk in the flesh, bro!"

Say what? *Um, you'll never find carne asada under my feet. I have a special file in my belly with its name on it.*

However, it didn't take long for me to master the meaning of the phrase. More importantly, I quickly began to identify the flesh in myself and to become intimately familiar with its ways and workings and how it truly is the enemy within.

Sworn Enemies

So then, what is this mysterious and seemingly ambiguous element that the Bible calls the flesh? How does it work? What are the pitfalls associated with it? And most importantly, how can we conquer it in our quest for sexual purity?

The best place to start is Galatians 5. Here Paul the Apostle described the operations of the flesh in clear detail while also giving us a greater understanding of the Spirit of God within us:

> I say then: Walk in the Spirit, and you shall not fulfill the
> lust of the flesh. For the flesh lusts against the Spirit, and
> the Spirit against the flesh; and these are contrary to one

another, so that you do not do the things that you wish. But if you are led by the Spirit, you are not under the law.

Now the works of the flesh are evident, which are: adultery, fornication, uncleanness, lewdness, idolatry, sorcery, hatred, contentions, jealousies, outbursts of wrath, selfish ambitions, dissensions, heresies, envy, murders, drunkenness, revelries, and the like; of which I tell you beforehand, just as I also told you in time past, that those who practice such things will not inherit the kingdom of God.

But the fruit of the Spirit is love, joy, peace, long-suffering, kindness, goodness, faithfulness, gentleness, self-control. Against such there is no law. And those who are Christ's have crucified the flesh with its passions and desires. If we live in the Spirit, let us also walk in the Spirit. Let us not become conceited, provoking one another, envying one another. (vv. 16–26)

Paul wasted no time acquainting his Galatian audience with the flesh—this element that he indicated is constantly at war with the Spirit of God. In juxtaposing these two realities that indwell the believer, Paul gave clear indicators that will help us contrast the operations of the flesh from the operations of the Spirit—through markers called works and fruit.

Relax—You're Not a Doomed Misfit

Before we do a deep dive into exploring the flesh and the Spirit, it's important to note the purpose behind the epic battle that is constantly raging between the two. Paul said that it's "so that you do not do the things that you wish" (v. 17). The "you" is in direct reference to the spiritually regenerated inner man, who always seeks to do what pleases the Lord. The battle is indicative of the real conflict within that is often a perplexing source of agitation for most believers.

Understanding this conflict between the flesh and the Spirit is integral to the pathway to victory. Peter alluded to the importance of not being caught off guard by certain types of trials or tests that we encounter as believers: "Beloved, do not think it strange concerning the fiery trial which is to try you, as though some strange thing happened to you" (1

Peter 4:12). Shock can often lead to confusion, confusion to disillusionment, and disillusionment to spiritual paralysis.

Do you recall the illustration I shared in chapter 1 about someone thinking they're headed for a luxury resort when they're really headed for a battlefield? Remember that how you perceive what's going on inside you will greatly impact your response. If you think that you're a misfit who's doomed to struggle with some sort of bizarre spiritual schizophrenia for the rest of your days, then you can be sure that you will experience much disappointment in your life. However, if you recognize that the tug-of-war inside you is a normal part of the Christian experience and one that God will cause to work together for good in your life as He conforms you to the image of Christ, then you will surely know joy and delight.

After Peter exhorted his embattled audience not to be surprised by their "fiery trial," he enlightened them to the type of mind-blowing alternative that is available for them: "Rejoice to the extent that you partake of Christ's sufferings, that when His glory is revealed, you may also be glad with exceeding joy" (v. 13).

"Rejoice" and "be glad with exceeding joy" are not the sorts of directives that we expect to see associated with trials and tribulation. While it's certain that most Christians are not naturally inclined to have a positive outlook on the flesh-Spirit dynamic, we should be heartened by the fact that God has outlined a clear pathway to victory for us in this struggle.

What in the World Is That Thing?

Now let's focus on this great enemy of ours—the flesh. The New Testament uses the word numerous times in this context, and it never appears in a positive light. The flesh is that part of our nature that was corrupted because of man's fall in Eden. It's an inherited reality that is diametrically opposed to righteousness and everything that is pleasing in the sight of God (Romans 5:12). Paul said as much when he thunderously declared, "I know that in me (that is, in my flesh) nothing good dwells" (7:18). And he didn't conceal the lethal ramifications associated with the flesh as he exclaimed this in the succeeding chapter: "If you live according to the flesh you will die" (8:13). The Greek word for "flesh," used in these two verses and in other key places throughout the epistles, is the word *sarx*. Here is a clear and fitting definition of this word for "flesh" from *A Greek-English Lexicon of the New Testament and Other Early Christian Literature*: "The physical body as functioning entity...in Paul's thought [especially], all parts of the body constitute a totality known as...flesh, which is dominated by sin to such a degree that wherever flesh is, all forms of sin are [likewise] present, and no good thing can live."[1]

Although the flesh continues to reside within the believer, the Spirit of God, who now also indwells man and who has quickened man's formerly dead spirit, gives him a new power over it. We exercise this power through what Paul described in Romans 8:1 as "walk[ing] in the Spirit." This is another one of those peculiar concepts that's somewhat difficult to comprehend. What in the world does it mean to walk in the Spirit? How do we do that?

The word for "walk" (in Greek *peripateō*) in its original context touches on the way one lives and conducts oneself.[2] It conveys the idea of being controlled by the Spirit of God in all areas of life. Nothing will more effectively help this reality materialize for a Christian than participating in the things that God's Spirit is involved in. And the highlight of Paul's exhortation is that walking in the Spirit is the way *not* to fulfill the lusts of the flesh. When our focus becomes walking in the Spirit, the strong pull to fulfill the lusts of the flesh will consequently weaken, and the flesh's power over us will diminish incrementally.

It's important to note here that among the various elements that Paul listed in connection with the works of the flesh, he included these crucial ones: "adultery, fornication, uncleanness, and lewdness." Paul then ended this descriptive list by saying, "and the like" (Galatians 5:19–21), which would include anything even slightly associated with these things. This demonstrates that sexual immorality of any kind is an undeniable work of the flesh. On the flip side, when enumerating the elements that make up the fruit of the Spirit, we find that Paul included goodness, faithfulness, and self-control. These undoubtedly apply to walking in sexual purity. As we walk in the Spirit and He controls us

1   Walter Bauer, *A Greek-English Lexicon of the New Testament and Other Early Christian Literature*, ed. Frederick Willian Danker, 3rd ed. (Chicago: University of Chicago Press, 2000), 915.
2   *Thayer's Expanded Greek Definition*, "Peripateō," StudyLight.org, accessed August 31, 2023, https://www.studylight.org.

to bear goodness, faithfulness, and self-control (see vv. 22–23), any sort of sexual immorality associated with adultery, fornication, uncleanness, lewdness, and the like will die off in our lives.

But again, the key is to immerse ourselves in the Spirit's activities. When we look at Scripture, we can identify four main things that the Holy Spirit is involved in: prayer, the Word of God, fellowship, and evangelism. When a Christian exercises active intentionality in all these various areas, it leads to close and intimate fellowship with the Spirit of God. This then creates a greater susceptibility for Him to control the believer. Let's now examine these four crucial areas that are indispensable to the Spirit-controlled life.

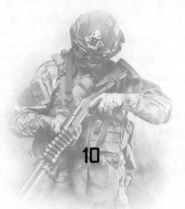

10

PRAYER

THE CHRISTIAN'S SPIRITUAL MORSE CODE

Can't Stop Hitting That Snooze Button

If we're honest with ourselves, we'll readily admit that prayer is one of the most challenging spiritual disciplines. We would much rather listen to a powerful sermon, engage in some soul-stirring fellowship, and sing our hearts out in corporate worship. But when it comes to prayer, we often find ourselves getting restless and our thoughts wandering away. And if we somehow manage to reign our roaming mind back in, we end up struggling to keep it awake.

If you can identify with this, rest assured that you're not alone. There's a reason why this is the common experience of every believer. It's definitely not a new battle, and we can see that even the original disciples fought to stay awake during prayer. The Bible tells us that when Jesus was in the garden of Gethsemane, just before He was arrested and crucified, He was "sorrowful and deeply distressed." In fact, He told His disciples that He was "sorrowful, even unto death" (Matthew 26:37–38).

Luke gives us deeper insight into the extent of Jesus' turmoil: "Being in agony, He prayed more earnestly. Then His sweat became like great drops of blood falling down to the ground" (22:44). Matthew tells us that Jesus took Peter, James, and John with Him and asked them to pray and watch with Him as He went a short distance from them to pour out His heart to the Father. Three times Jesus returned to them, and each time He found them asleep. After He came to them the first time, He said something very insightful to Peter: "What! Could you not watch with Me one hour? Watch and pray, lest you enter into temptation. The spirit indeed is willing, but the flesh is weak" (Matthew 26:40–41).

Here we see the faithful trio—the ragtag disciples. They were the select few the Savior handpicked to be His chosen ones, companions, apostles. There were others, of course, but these few were the inner circle of the inner circle, and on this particular occasion, Jesus specifically tapped them to be with Him in His intense hour of trial. Of course, they desired to honor their Savior, to answer the call, to back Him up, and to intercede for Him on that dark, foreboding night. Everything within their spirit was willing, but their flesh was weak. Yes, the flesh is indeed weak, weaker than we typically realize, especially when it comes to prayer.

Beefing Up Your Barometer Reading

I believe that the quality of a Christian's prayer life is a barometer indicating how they're doing spiritually. Prayer, being as challenging as it sometimes is and requiring a reasonable measure of faith, is not the sort of activity that spiritually anemic believers usually engage in. In fact, the lack of prayer in a person's life is often the primary cause of their spiritual anemia. It's a catch-22 of sorts. Kind of the opposite of perpetual motion, it's almost like perpetual degeneration. People become spiritually anemic by not engaging in prayer, and when they're spiritually anemic, it becomes all the more difficult for them to engage in prayer. Setting aside time daily to commune with a God whose face we cannot see, whose voice we cannot hear, and whose presence we cannot physically feel is a good indicator of vibrant faith in the life of a Christian. And this is especially true when the prayers include selfless intercession for others and a pleading for God's will to be done in the world.

John Bunyan, the famous Puritan who gave the world *The Pilgrim's Progress*, one of the best-selling and most cherished books of all time, understood the value of prayer as he endured twelve years in prison because of his faith in Christ. His exhortation is both sobering and encouraging: "You can do more than pray after you have prayed, but you cannot do more than pray until you have prayed. Pray often, for prayer is a shield to the soul, a sacrifice to God, and a scourge to Satan."[1]

It's important to note, however, that while prayer undoubtedly unleashes spiritual vitality in a Christian's life, a very practical component is the driving force behind it. It's very simple yet profound. God hears the cries of His people, and He answers them. We have real needs and so do others, and we have a sovereign, loving God who has the power to address those needs in keeping with what's best for us and those for whom we intercede. And His Word very clearly tells us that sometimes we have not because we ask not (James 4:2). This means that God conditions certain provisions in our lives on our prayers and petitions.

When it comes to the practical effectiveness of prayer in our battle against sexual sin, Jesus' words to Peter, James, and John in Gethsemane could not be clearer. He said in Matthew 26:41, "Watch and pray, lest you enter into temptation." This coincides with the prayer model that He passed on to them in what has been famously called the Lord's Prayer (though it is really the Christian's prayer, which the Lord taught to His disciples): "Do not lead us into temptation, but deliver us from the evil one" (6:13).

He-Man Got It Wrong—Jesus Has the Power

One of the most common words we often use alongside the word *prayer* is *power*. The world is full of resources that tout "the power of prayer." While I realize that this is often a simple matter of semantics, the words we use can definitely impact our outlook and our behavior. Rather than highlight the power of prayer, I think it would be better to focus on the power of God to answer prayer.

If we're led to believe that our prayers themselves possess power, then when we're lacking focus or energy or desire or enthusiasm or even the "right" words, we're prone to become discouraged and conclude that prayer is powerless. This will, in turn, make us less inclined to persevere in prayer. But suppose our focus is on our almighty, omnipotent God, who spans the universe with His hand, who has sovereign control over every atom in the universe, and for whom nothing is impossible. Then, the consciousness of our own feebleness against the backdrop of

1   John Bunyan, *Prayer* (Carlisle, PA: Banner of Truth, 1999), 23.

such a powerful God who loves us will make us more eager to pour out our hearts to Him, knowing that He hears our faintest whispers and can move mountains and galaxies to fulfill His will in our lives.

Cracking the Confidence Code

While God's power should be the focal point that motivates our supplications, there is a particular benefit that His power provides us *through* prayer that should fill our hearts with rapturous joy. This benefit is called confidence: "This is the confidence that we have in Him, that if we ask anything according to His will, He hears us. And if we know that He hears us, whatever we ask, we know that we have the petitions that we have asked of Him" (1 John 5:14–15).

Few qualities in this world are more liberating for a Christian than confidence. It creates a deep sense of security in the believer. Security then gives way to peace. Peace, in turn, creates an occasion for freedom, and freedom results in us becoming a completely surrendered and useful instrument in the hand of God. John told us that the confidence that triggers this whole glorious domino effect is rooted in the knowledge that God hears us whenever we ask for things that are in keeping with His will. Chew on that for a minute. The infinite God of the universe actually hears your voice when you cry out to Him. But we are not meant to understand the hearing that John was referring to as literal hearing. We know that God hears all things and that nothing has ever escaped the reach of His divine ears. We are to understand this hearing as God taking notice of your request with the intention of fulfilling it. He fulfills it because it aligns with His will, and this is why John concluded by saying that "if we know that He hears us, whatever we ask, we know that we have the petitions that we have asked of Him" (v. 15).

But an implied confidence is available to us on the flip side of this reality. If we ask for something that's not in keeping with God's will, He will not take notice of our request with the intention of fulfilling it. Instead, after taking notice of it, He determines to deny our request. This is because it doesn't coincide with His divine will for our lives, which means it's not best for our good and His glory. And if something is not in keeping with God's will for our lives, no matter how badly we may think we want it, ultimately, it's the last thing we really want.

FIGHT LIKE A MAN

So whether God says yes or no to our prayers, once we have prayed, we should experience the benefits of confidence, security, peace, freedom, and, ultimately, the pleasure and honor of being useful to the Lord. This should give us a whole new perspective on prayer when we read Paul's words in Philippians 4:6–7, where he exhorted us to put off anxiousness and to make our requests known to God. It should thrill us to no end when we read that we should pray without ceasing (1 Thessalonians 5:17), cast our cares upon Him (1 Peter 5:7), and continue earnestly in prayer, being vigilant in it with thanksgiving (Colossians 4:2).

It's Yours for the Asking

While an active prayer life, generally speaking, is indispensable to walking in the Spirit and, therefore, a deterrent to giving in to the lusts of the flesh, the confidence God provides through prayer should motivate us to pray specifically for victory over sexual temptations. And we can do this with complete assurance that these sorts of prayers are in keeping with God's will because His Word tells us they are: "This is the will of God, your sanctification: that you should abstain from sexual immorality" (1 Thessalonians 4:3).

If we know that God gives us an open invitation to cast our burdens at His feet, that it's His will for us to abstain from sexual immorality, and that He always answers prayers that are in keeping with His will, then how eager should we be to regularly cry out to Him for help with our sexual struggles? The key is to pray not only when the temptations are raging but also when we don't sense any temptations at all. This is the epitome of building up the type of preventive preparedness we discussed earlier in this book. These are what we might call preventative prayers. They are in keeping with Christ's petition: "Do not lead into temptation" (Matthew 6:13). In this vein, J. C. Ryle, in his riveting book *A Call to Prayer*, said this: "Praying and sinning will never live together in the same heart. Prayer will consume sin, or sin will choke prayer."[2]

---

2   J. C. Ryle, *A Call to Prayer* (Pensacola, FL: Mount Zion Bible Institute, 1998), 8, https://www.chapellibrary.org.

PRAYER

Help for the Helpless from the Helping Helper

In John 14 and 16, Jesus spoke of the Holy Spirit coming into the lives of believers after His departure from them. He referred to the Holy Spirit as the *Paraclete* in the Greek. That word translates to "Helper," "Advocate," "Comforter," and "Counselor." All those words are so fitting, and they perfectly describe the Spirit's divine activity in the life of the Christian. It's a joy to know that the Spirit's help, advocacy, comfort, and counsel are all available to us in the arena of prayer: "Likewise the Spirit also helps in our weaknesses. For we do not know what we should pray for as we ought, but the Spirit Himself makes intercession for us with groanings which cannot be uttered" (Romans 8:26).

J. C. Ryle's words once more add vivid color to this biblical truth: "The Spirit will give us words if we seek His aid. The prayers of the Lord's people are the inspiration of the Lord's Spirit, the work of the Holy Ghost who dwells within them as the Spirit of grace and supplication."[3]

Not only does the Holy Spirit assist us in the content of our prayers, but He also helps to infuse us with the animating strength to pray, as R. Kent Hughes so aptly wrote, "[Another] benefit of praying in the Spirit is that it supplies the energizing of the Holy Spirit for prayer, infusing tired, even infirm, bodies and elevating the depressed to pray with power and conviction."[4]

In an influential book on the subject of prayer, an unknown Christian author expounded something that I believe resonates with every lover of Christ: "Why are many Christians so often defeated? Because they pray so little. Why are many church-workers so often discouraged and disheartened? Because they pray so little. Why do most men see so few brought 'out of darkness to light' by their ministry? Because they pray so little. Why are not our churches simply on fire for God? Because there is so little real prayer...We may be assured of this: the secret of all failure is our failure in secret prayer."[5]

He went on to say, "Do we realize that there is nothing the devil dreads so much as prayer? His great concern is to keep us from praying. He loves to see us 'up to our eyes' in work, provided we do not pray.

---

3   Ryle, *A Call to Prayer*, 9.
4   R. Kent Hughes, *Disciplines of a Godly Man*, updated ed. (Wheaton, IL: Crossway, 2019), 123.
5   *The Kneeling Christian* (Grand Rapids, MI: Zondervan, 1986), 14.

He does not fear because we are eager and earnest Bible students, provided we are little in prayer. Someone has wisely said, 'Satan laughs at our toiling, mocks at our wisdom, but trembles when we pray.'"[6]

May you be determined to proactively walk in the Spirit as you engage with Him through a powerful and revolutionary prayer life.

---

6   *The Kneeling Christian*, 18.

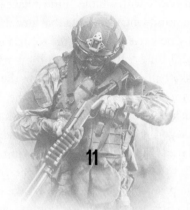

11

GOD'S WORD

THE BELIEVER'S EXCALIBUR

This Boy Needs *The Bible for Dummies* Book

I grew up somewhat understanding that the Bible is God's Word, but I never read much of it—and I definitely didn't understand what it was really all about. When my family moved to a new neighborhood during my seventh-grade year, I quickly became friends with another teenager on my street who grew up in a Christian home. He wasn't quite walking the straight and narrow at the time, so he would lie to his parents and tell them that he was coming over to my house (the new heathen on the block) to do a Bible study with me. But of course, the only thing we had planned to study was the life of two famous brothers who were Super Saints—Mario and Luigi—out of the epistle of First Nintendoians.

Yeah, I know, pretty scandalous. But it gets worse. The first time my friend came over for a reverent time of "Bible study," I happened to be in the front yard as he was walking up toward my house. I immediately saw his Bible in his hand and nearly had a panic attack. I remember thinking, *This isn't going to fly.* But I came up with a quick solution and said, "Hey, can you put your Bible in my mailbox? My parents will think it's very weird if you come into our house with a Bible." I must have been the wretch that John Newton had in mind when he wrote that amazing hymn.

Eventually, my new friend invited me to start going to his church's midweek service with him. Sitting through the boring Bible study was painful, but the basketball games we played after the services sure made the torture a little more tolerable. I was positive the Bible must have said something like, "Basketball is next to godliness." That would have made me one of the world's godliest kids because I definitely loved basketball—and we certainly played a lot of it at my friend's church.

I'll never forget the first time I attended the youth group meeting with my buddy. The pastor asked everyone to take out their Bibles and then instructed us to turn to a specific section. It was the book of something or other, chapter such and such, and verse this or that. *Huh?* I remember feeling completely lost and embarrassed as all the kids around me effortlessly flicked through their Bibles, and I recall distinctly saying to myself, *I will never learn how to use a Bible.*

Who would have ever guessed that after a few years, I would find myself as a biblical studies major in college, later becoming an ordained pastor and Bible teacher, and currently leading a Christian ministry that has a foundation built on God's Word. But the most divinely comical thing of all is that I have the privilege of serving as the host and spokesperson for the National Bible Bee Competition. Only God!

Profiting from God's Word

As I'm sure you've lightly surmised by now, I'm a passionate lover of the Holy Bible. I will unashamedly admit, however, that it's all about the profit for me. Yes, it's true; my real motive is to profit from God's Word. But more importantly, that's exactly what God wants for me, and profit is what He designed His Word to produce for me—and for you: "All Scripture is given by inspiration of God, and is profitable for doctrine, for reproof, for correction, for instruction in righteousness, that the man of God may be complete, thoroughly equipped for every good work" (2 Timothy 3:16–17).

As a Christian, those words are music to my ears. To be spiritually complete and thoroughly equipped is the dream of every eternally minded and eternally invested child of God. Scripture makes it clear that this is the ultimate profit that God's Word supplies as it establishes us in solid doctrine while reproving us, correcting us, and instructing us in righteousness.

The Love Boat Gone Wrong

So why is 2 Timothy 3:16–17 important? Because, as we discovered a few chapters ago, it coincides with and makes possible one of the most crucial aspects of our very existence, which we read about in 2 Corinthians 5:9: "We make it our aim, whether present or absent, to be well pleasing to Him."

If our aim in life is to be well pleasing to the Lord, does it not logically follow that we need to know what He has clearly declared is well pleasing to Him? And where else can we find those things clearly declared but in His inspired, inerrant, infallible Word? If the lighthouse of God's glorious Word does not guide us through the dark and perilous seas of life, then we will be like ships lost in the ocean of uncertainty, hopelessly adrift with no motor, rudder, oar, sail, or compass—inevitably headed toward shipwreck on the merciless rocks of this world's folly.

A good rule of thumb to remember during this brief breath that we call life is that if we don't rely on God's Word to direct us, we will have no other recourse but to look to our own human reasoning, which will often lead us astray because it flows from a fallen and depraved nature.

Without God's Wisdom, We's Dumb

Imagine what life must be like for someone who professes to be a Christian but does not have an intimate knowledge of the Bible's contents. As this man goes through the normal course of life, he will inevitably face circumstances that demand a decision between opposing choices. If he lacks the wisdom of God's Word, the only guide for his reasoning will be the brand of worldly wisdom that will almost certainly lead him in the wrong direction. Here are a few different scenarios in that vein:

He meets the woman of his dreams, and everything lines up perfectly. He loves her looks, her personality, her sense of humor, and her moral standards. They have amazing chemistry together, similar goals and aspirations in life, and the same pet peeves. They even hang their toilet paper roll the same way. However, this amazing woman is not a

Christian. Now worldly wisdom would ask, *And what's the problem?* In fact, most non-Christians would reprimand the believer for having even the slightest hesitation to pursue such a relationship and would cry discrimination. But if a man knows what is pleasing to God through His Word, then he would realize that a long-term relationship with this woman is a definite no-go because Scripture clearly forbids it:

> Do not be unequally yoked together with unbelievers.
> For what fellowship has righteousness with lawlessness?
> And what communion has light with darkness? And what
> accord has Christ with Belial? Or what part has a believer
> with an unbeliever? And what agreement has the temple of
> God with idols? For you are the temple of the living God.
> As God has said:
> "I will dwell in them
> and walk among them.
> I will be their God,
> and they shall be My people."
> Therefore
> "Come out from among them
> and be separate, says the Lord.
> Do not touch what is unclean,
> and I will receive you."
> "I will be a Father to you,
> and you shall be My sons and daughters,
> says the LORD Almighty." (2 Corinthians 6:14–18)

It would seem logical to any rational, thinking person that God would never want His people to pay taxes to a government that supports such things as abortion, gay marriage, and transgenderism. However, God has a different perspective on the matter. And remember, the following things were written in the context of a Roman government that was not only oppressive but also supportive of and mired in grotesque immorality:

> They sent to Him some of the Pharisees and the Herodians,
> to catch Him in His words. When they had come, they

said to Him, "Teacher, we know that You are true, and care about no one; for You do not regard the person of men, but teach the way of God in truth. Is it lawful to pay taxes to Caesar, or not? Shall we pay, or shall we not pay?"

But He, knowing their hypocrisy, said to them, "Why do you test Me? Bring Me a denarius that I may see it." So they brought it.

And He said to them, "Whose image and inscription is this?" They said to Him, "Caesar's."

And Jesus answered and said to them, "Render to Caesar the things that are Caesar's, and to God the things that are God's."

And they marveled at Him. (Mark 12:13–17)

Elsewhere, Scripture says, "Because of this you also pay taxes, for they are God's ministers attending continually to this very thing. Render therefore to all their due: taxes to whom taxes are due, customs to whom customs, fear to whom fear, honor to whom honor" (Romans 13:6–7).

While Christians generally understand that wives are called to be submissive toward their husbands, no one would think that Jesus would want a woman to submit to a man who is not walking in obedience to His Word. Or would He?

Wives, likewise, be submissive to your own husbands, that even if some do not obey the word, they, without a word, may be won by the conduct of their wives, when they observe your chaste conduct accompanied by fear. Do not let your adornment be merely outward—arranging the hair, wearing gold, or putting on fine apparel—rather let it be the hidden person of the heart, with the incorruptible beauty of a gentle and quiet spirit, which is very precious in the sight of God. For in this manner, in former times, the holy women who trusted in God also adorned themselves, being submissive to their own husbands, as Sarah obeyed Abraham, calling him lord, whose daughters you are if you do good and are not afraid with any terror. (1 Peter 3:1–6)

It's important to note here that Scripture in no way calls a woman to submit to abuse. And the Bible does not call her to submit when her husband asks her to do anything that violates God's Word. In general, we are always to submit to those who have official authority over us (within the context of their jurisdiction) unless they are being abusive, are commanding us to do something God forbids, or are forbidding us to do something God commands.

When it comes to the tone and tenor of relationships between those who profess to know Christ, it only makes sense that we do everything possible to keep those who are living unrepentant lives within the confines of the church. After all, maintaining close ties with them will create opportunities for them to continue to hear truth, increasing their chances of getting right with God. But is this what God prescribed?

> I wrote to you in my epistle not to keep company with sexually immoral people. Yet I certainly did not mean with the sexually immoral people of this world, or with the covetous, or extortioners, or idolaters, since then you would need to go out of the world. But now I have written to you not to keep company with anyone named a brother, who is sexually immoral, or covetous, or an idolater, or a reviler, or a drunkard, or an extortioner—not even to eat with such a person.
>
> For what have I to do with judging those also who are outside? Do you not judge those who are inside? But those who are outside God judges. Therefore "put away from yourselves the evil person." (1 Corinthians 5:9–13)

I hope that these few examples have given you a glimpse into why it's critical for every Christian to become intimately familiar with Scripture. It's the only objective standard by which we can know, with certainty, what is pleasing to the Lord. And it's indisputable that the Holy Spirit is actively involved in the Bible because we're told that the Word of God is the "sword of the Spirit" (Ephesians 6:17). In fact, the book of Hebrews makes it clear that Scripture is mightier than any earthly sword that has ever been wielded: "The word of God is living and powerful, and sharper than any two-edged sword, piercing even to the division of soul and spirit, and of joints and marrow, and is a discerner of the thoughts and intents of the heart" (4:12).

Bein' a Berean and Searchin' and Seein'

In order to experience the full power of God's Word in our lives, we must do more than just read it. We need to follow the example of a group of Jews in the book of Acts called the Bereans: "These were more fair-minded than those in Thessalonica, in that they received the word with all readiness, and searched the Scriptures daily to find out whether these things were so" (17:11).

When these Bereans heard Paul and Silas proclaim the Word, they did not have a nonchalant attitude about it. Instead, they received it with great eagerness. But after they enthusiastically received it, they then researched it to be sure that what they had heard was true.

A Shifting Shack or a Shiftless Château

Along with the decision to receive and research the Word, there is one more indispensable step that people must take to experience the Bible's full impact—and that crucial step is to respond to it. We're not meant just to know and admire the Scriptures; we're called to act on them.

This coincides with what we're exhorted to do in the book of James: "Be doers of the word, and not hearers only, deceiving yourselves" (1:22).

And Jesus didn't mince any words when He spoke about what would be experienced by those who know but don't do His Word:

Whoever hears these sayings of Mine, and does them, I will liken him to a wise man who built his house on the rock: and the rain descended, the floods came, and the winds blew and beat on that house; and it did not fall, for it was founded on the rock.

But everyone who hears these sayings of Mine, and does not do them, will be like a foolish man who built his house on the sand: and the rain descended, the floods came, and the winds blew and beat on that house; and it fell. And great was its fall. (Matthew 7:24–27)

FIGHT LIKE A MAN

If someone decides to receive, research, and respond to God's Word, then regardless of their circumstances in life, they will experience its transformative power. If they're an unbeliever, God's Word will reveal to them the truth that will require a response of either receiving or rejecting the person of Christ. If they've strayed from the faith, it will cause them to realize their folly, repent, recommit, and be restored. If they're going through doubts and trials, God's Word will reassure them of their salvation, reaffirm God's love for them, and remind them to rejoice in tribulation. If they're going through a slump or a dry spell, it will revive, renew, rejuvenate, and reinvigorate them. And if they're walking in the Spirit, God's Word will spark refreshment and rejoicing. This is because the Word of God is His radical, remarkable, reliable, reasonable, readable, revolutionary revelation, and it will not return to Him void.

Money Doesn't Grow *on* Trees But...

Since becoming a Christian back in 1991, I've had the privilege of experiencing the priceless benefits of God's Word in countless ways. The Bible guides and guards me, strengthens and soothes me, convicts and compels me, enlightens and encourages me—all the while informing and instructing me in every aspect of my life. I'm often saddened when I consider the fact that those who don't know Christ are left without the Maker's divine instruction manual to navigate the complexities of this world and figure out how everything is supposed to work.

We live in an era where many profess to greatly value truth. It seems that most are frantically and incessantly searching for it in every direction. The sad thing is that the fullness of truth is right beneath their nose in the treasure house of God's Word, and they don't even realize it.

Many years ago, when I served as an associate pastor of a local church, we launched a men's school of ministry through which we planned to train young men to serve the cause of Christ—both domestically and on the mission field. To do this effectively, we needed to find a home to rent that was spacious enough to house multiple students and staff members. We also needed a sizable piece of property since we intended to teach these students construction skills so that they could one day pursue tent-making jobs while ministering, if necessary. After much searching, we finally found exactly what we were looking for. The only problem was that the two-acre property was a cross between a dump and a junkyard. Amid the mountains of garbage, we found an old car, a bathtub, and at least ninety thousand toilets (maybe I'm exaggerating about finding a bathtub). After multiple workdays and what seemed like countless man-hours, we finally finished clearing the land. We then turned our attention toward landscaping. Of all the trees on the property (and there were many), we found only one that we decided to remove because it was an obstacle.

After our team cut the tree down, some of the self-professed lumberjacks of the bunch gave the crew a lecture on how to properly remove the remaining trunk. The men began enthusiastically implementing their newfound knowledge by digging a trench around the trunk and pouring water into it to loosen up the roots and finally yank it out.

In the process of digging the trench—as the pickax penetrated the soil—they heard the sound of breaking glass. They looked down and were utterly shocked to find wads of cash sticking out of the ground. It was $50 million! Just kidding. It was actually $2,200 packed inside that buried jar, but that was nothing to sneeze at because the bills dated back to the 1930s. At that time in history, you could buy a brand-new car for $700. The average annual income was about $1,300. There were even some places in the United States where you could buy a home in the $3,000 range. So back in that time, $2,200 was a massive treasure. The person who first said, "Money doesn't grow on trees," was right—he just forgot to look under them.

I couldn't help but wonder how many residents of that property over the course of decades had sat on that very spot—perhaps weeping about their financial woes—when right beneath their nose was a massive treasure. There's only one thing that's more tragic than having a treasure within reach and not knowing it: it's knowing where the treasure is but never digging it out and experiencing the benefits of its riches. While the world may not know about the priceless gems and jewels of truth within the precious Word of God, as believers, we do know about them. How passionate should we then be about diligently mining those truths and allowing them to transform us?

Soul Food

It's high time that Christian men finally grasp the fact that integrating God's Word into their lives is an indispensable component to achieving victory over sexual sin. Psalm 119 makes this abundantly clear: "How can a young man cleanse his way? By taking heed according to Your word" (v. 9). Another translation gives us an even clearer understanding of what the psalmist intended to convey: "How can a young man keep his way pure? By keeping it according to Your word" (NASB). A couple of verses later in the same psalm, we find this inspiring truth: "Your word I have hidden in my heart, that I might not sin against You" (v. 11).

So if we're intent on keeping our way pure and not sinning against the Lord by participating in sexual immorality, then we must take heed to God's Word and hide it in our heart. We do this by being determined to faithfully read the Bible every day. To harken back to the Bereans, this is one of the ways that we receive the Word with great eagerness. There are loads of one-year Bible reading plans that we can go through. There are also countless books, video courses, websites, and apps that can enhance our reading of Scripture and help us implement effective strategies to intake more of God's divine revelation.[1]

Even the Unstudious Will Study This

Along with having a daily reading plan, we also need to be determined to study the Scriptures and ensure that we understand what we're reading. Again, like our forerunners in Berea, this is how we examine (or research) the Scriptures. There are great books that can help you learn how to properly interpret the Bible (a study called hermeneutics). Also lots of commentaries and online sermons, written and preached by godly men, will exposit or explain what the Scriptures mean in their proper context.

Memo-rise and Shine

One of the things I'm extremely passionate about in life is memorizing Scripture. This has been one of the most fruitful spiritual disciplines I've ever engaged in. While studying God's Word is foundational, locking

---

1   For those looking for resources, Ray Comfort's *My Comfort Is Jesus* contains an excellent one-year Bible reading plan, and if you want a powerful study Bible that will inspire you to read more of Scripture, check out *The Evidence Study Bible*, compiled by Ray Comfort.

the verses we've studied into our hearts and minds will give us constant access to those truths. And access to the sword of the Spirit when we're in the heat of battle fighting temptations is paramount to victory over those temptations. Having the best sword in the world is wonderful, but it doesn't do you any good if it's sitting at home in its scabbard while an enemy attacks you on the battlefield. To be doers of God's Word (or responders to it), its truths must constantly inform our hearts and minds in real time.

Memorizing Scripture can often feel quite daunting. But if you start small and build your way up, you'll be amazed by your brain's capacity to capture and recall what you feed it. By God's grace, I'm currently close to memorizing more than half of the books of the New Testament (I'm presently working on book fourteen out of twenty-seven). This has taken me years, but there was a day when my adventure began with the first word of the first verse of the first chapter of the first book. Soon I'll be close to having memorized fifty chapters and nearly one thousand verses. Sometimes it shocks me when I really think about it. But as the old saying goes, "The journey of a thousand miles begins with a first step."

While I'm not immune to becoming prideful about this accomplishment (which would contradict the whole purpose of memorizing God's Word), the one thing that keeps my pride in check is thinking about the amazing young people I've worked with from the National Bible Bee Competition (NBBC). As I said, it has taken me many, many years to memorize almost one thousand verses, but some of these teenagers have memorized that many verses over the course of one summer—yes, one single summer! And then they stand on a stage in front of a watching audience and must instantly recite (word-perfect) long passages of Scripture that the judges present to them at lightning speed. No pressure there at all.

If you're reading this book and you happen to be a young man in your teen years (thirteen to eighteen), I encourage you to speak with your parents about the possibility of participating in the NBBC. You don't have to compete at the national level; there are local summer competitions that are less rigorous but extremely valuable in helping you memorize God's Word. Visit BibleBee.org to learn more.

But whether you're a teenager or not, you're blessed to live in a day and age where helpful resources abound and are easily accessible. Just as books, study courses, videos, podcasts, online articles, and apps can help you study the Bible, these same mediums can also help you grow in memorizing Scripture. Don't put this off. Tap into these resources and get started today.

For More than Just Misguided and Muttering Mystics

After you consistently read, study, and memorize God's Word, there is one more crucial and revolutionary spiritual discipline that will help shape you into an obedient man of God, into the type of man who has his house built on the rock rather than on the sand, into the one that Jesus said will not fall when the storms of life blow your way. I'm talking about meditating on Scripture.

Meditation is not a very popular practice among Christians. We give it lip service from time to time but don't really integrate it into the rhythm of our lives. I wonder if this is perhaps due to subconsciously associating it with Eastern mysticism or New Age practices. But rest assured that meditation is a very biblical and beneficial practice. In fact, the book of Psalms introduces us to its significance in the first few verses of its opening chapter:

> Blessed is the man
> who walks not in the counsel of the ungodly,
> nor stands in the path of sinners,
> nor sits in the seat of the scornful;
> but his delight is in the law of the LORD,
> and in His law he meditates day and night.
> He shall be like a tree
> planted by the rivers of water,
> that brings forth its fruit in its season,
> whose leaf also shall not wither;
> and whatever he does shall prosper. (1:1–3)

The biblical concept of meditating on God's law (or Word) that Psalm 1 conveys is related to the methodical way a cow feeds on grass. It involves chewing it, then swallowing it, regurgitating it, chewing it again, and then swallowing it once more. The cow repeats this process until its body fully absorbs all the nutrients. When it comes to God's Word, meditation involves muttering truth to yourself and letting it ruminate in your heart and mind until it becomes fully integrated into your very being. And the outcome will be stability, fruitfulness, endurance, and spiritual prosperity.

Never in the course of human history has the mind of man been bombarded with more relentless distractions than it is now. With countless electronic devices; rapidly multiplying social media platforms; limitless access to websites, video games, movies, blogs, vlogs, apps, articles, videos, and so much more, it's hard for our brains to ever get any peace and quiet. Thinking has almost become a lost art because incessant noise rules the day. We simply don't know how to sit still in silence anymore. And what a shame. But those who regularly will themselves into that serene and contemplative mode of meditation on God's Word—despite being hounded by resistant emotions—will experience a divine strength that will deepen their roots in the Lord unlike anything else.

The world understands how indispensable solitude and meditation are for success in the business arena. Though an unquestionably controversial figure, Bill Gates, the billionaire founder of Microsoft, established a habit of getting away for a weeklong, private retreat twice each year. He dubbed these crucial escapes "Think Weeks." A seaplane or helicopter would drop him off at a secret cabin somewhere in a remote Pacific Northwest forest. Very few people knew where he was, and no one was allowed to visit. Contact with others was limited to someone delivering two meals to him daily. Bill Gates would spend focused time—on some days, up to eighteen hours—reading pertinent corporate documents and intensively thinking through them. Some of Microsoft's most successful initiatives originated during these special retreats. The alone-time concept became so valuable to his corporation that Gates prescribed it to their top fifty engineering thinkers. No wonder Microsoft remains one of the world's most dominant and lucrative companies.[2] Imagine what would happen if every Christian did this with God's Word, in miniature form, for even just fifteen minutes each day.

Going All Gideon on You

I hope that this chapter has whet your appetite for Holy Scripture and that you have become convicted in the very core of your being to make God's Word the foundation upon which you build your life. One Christian organization that has been faithfully committed to distributing God's Word across the globe, perhaps more than any other, is the Gideons International. If you ever stay in hotel rooms, you may, at some point, find one of their Bibles in a nightstand drawer. I absolutely love this powerful description of the Bible that they have included in many of their print runs of the Word:

> The Bible contains the mind of God, the state of man, the way of salvation, the doom of sinners, and the happiness of believers. Its doctrines are holy, its precepts are binding, its histories are true, and its decisions are immutable.
>
> Read it to be wise, believe it to be safe, and practice it to be holy. It contains light to direct you, food to support you, and comfort to cheer you.
>
> It is the traveler's map, the pilgrim's staff, the pilot's compass, the soldier's sword, and the Christian's charter. Here too, Heaven is opened and the gates of Hell disclosed.
>
> Christ is its grand subject, our good its design, and the glory of God its end. It should fill the memory, rule the heart, and guide the feet. Read it slowly, frequently, and prayerfully. It is a mine of wealth, a paradise of glory, and a river of pleasure.
>
> It is given you in life, will be opened at the judgment, and be remembered forever. It involves the highest responsibility, rewards the greatest labor, and will condemn all who trifle with its sacred contents.

---

2   Catherine Clifford, "Bill Gates Took Solo 'Think Weeks' in a Cabin in the Woods—Why It's a Great Strategy," CNBC, July 28, 2019, https://www.cnbc.com.

Armed with Ample Ammo for Your Artillery

To be a well-rounded Christian, it's imperative that you immerse yourself in the whole counsel of God and let all the contents of the sixty-six divinely inspired books of the Old and New Testaments inform every aspect of your life. However, as a man who is seeking to grow in sexual purity, it's also wise and fitting for you to read, study, memorize, and meditate on specific Scripture passages that are directly applicable to this topic—all in the spirit of seeking to receive, research, and respond in the affirmative to the Word of God. With this in mind, I will include some (and there are many more) key passages that will help to strengthen you and fortify your resolve in the pursuit of purity.

> You have heard that it was said to those of old, "You shall not commit adultery." But I say to you that whoever looks at a woman to lust for her has already committed adultery with her in her heart. If your right eye causes you to sin, pluck it out and cast it from you; for it is more profitable for you that one of your members perish, than for your whole body to be cast into hell. And if your right hand causes you to sin, cut it off and cast it from you; for it is more profitable for you that one of your members perish, than for your whole body to be cast into hell. (Matthew 5:27–30)

> Likewise you also, reckon yourselves to be dead indeed to sin, but alive to God in Christ Jesus our Lord.
> Therefore do not let sin reign in your mortal body, that you should obey it in its lusts. And do not present your members as instruments of unrighteousness to sin, but present yourselves to God as being alive from the dead, and your members as instruments of righteousness to God. For sin shall not have dominion over you, for you are not under law but under grace. (Romans 6:11–14)

> The night is far spent, the day is at hand. Therefore let us cast off the works of darkness, and let us put on the armor

of light. Let us walk properly, as in the day, not in revelry and drunkenness, not in lewdness and lust, not in strife and envy. But put on the Lord Jesus Christ, and make no provision for the flesh, to fulfill its lusts. (Romans 13:12–14)

Foods for the stomach and the stomach for foods, but God will destroy both it and them. Now the body is not for sexual immorality but for the Lord, and the Lord for the body. (1 Corinthians 6:13)

Flee sexual immorality. Every sin that a man does is outside the body, but he who commits sexual immorality sins against his own body. Or do you not know that your body is the temple of the Holy Spirit who is in you, whom you have from God, and you are not your own? For you were bought at a price; therefore glorify God in your body and in your spirit, which are God's. (1 Corinthians 6:18–20)

No temptation has overtaken you except such as is common to man; but God is faithful, who will not allow you to be tempted beyond what you are able, but with the temptation will also make the way of escape, that you may be able to bear it. (1 Corinthians 10:13)

Do not be deceived, God is not mocked; for whatever a man sows, that he will also reap. For he who sows to his flesh will of the flesh reap corruption, but he who sows to the Spirit will of the Spirit reap everlasting life. (Galatians 6:7–8)

Fornication and all uncleanness or covetousness, let it not even be named among you, as is fitting for saints; neither filthiness, nor foolish talking, nor coarse jesting, which are not fitting, but rather giving of thanks. For this you know, that no fornicator, unclean person, nor covetous man, who is an idolater, has any inheritance in the kingdom of Christ and God. Let no one deceive you with empty words, for because of these things the wrath of God comes upon the sons of disobedience. Therefore do not be partakers with them. (Ephesians 5:3–7)

Therefore put to death your members which are on the earth: fornication, uncleanness, passion, evil desire, and covetousness, which is idolatry. (Colossians 3:5)

This is the will of God, your sanctification: that you should abstain from sexual immorality; that each of you should know how to possess his own vessel in sanctification and honor, not in passion of lust, like the Gentiles who do not know God. (1 Thessalonians 4:3–5)

Flee also youthful lusts; but pursue righteousness, faith, love, peace with those who call on the Lord out of a pure heart. (2 Timothy 2:22)

We do not have a High Priest who cannot sympathize with our weaknesses, but was in all points tempted as we are, yet without sin. Let us therefore come boldly to the throne of grace, that we may obtain mercy and find grace to help in time of need. (Hebrews 4:15–16)

Let no one say when he is tempted, "I am tempted by God"; for God cannot be tempted by evil, nor does He Himself tempt anyone. But each one is tempted when he is drawn away by his own desires and enticed. Then, when desire has conceived, it gives birth to sin; and sin, when it is full-grown, brings forth death. (James 1:13–15)

How can a young man cleanse his way?
By taking heed according to Your word. (Psalm 119:9)

Your word I have hidden in my heart,
that I might not sin against You. (Psalm 119:11)

FIGHT LIKE A MAN

Let your eyes look straight ahead,
and your eyelids look right before you.
Ponder the path of your feet,
and let all your ways be established.
Do not turn to the right or the left;
remove your foot from evil. (Proverbs 4:25–27)

Can a man take fire to his bosom,
and his clothes not be burned?
Can one walk on hot coals,
and his feet not be seared?
So is he who goes in to his neighbor's wife;
whoever touches her shall not be innocent.
(Proverbs 6:27–29)

Whoever commits adultery with a woman lacks understanding;
he who does so destroys his own soul.
Wounds and dishonor he will get,
and his reproach will not be wiped away. (Proverbs 6:32–33)

For at the window of my house
I looked through my lattice,
and saw among the simple,
I perceived among the youths,
a young man devoid of understanding,
passing along the street near her corner;
and he took the path to her house
in the twilight, in the evening,
in the black and dark night.
And there a woman met him,
with the attire of a harlot, and a crafty heart.
She was loud and rebellious,
her feet would not stay at home.
At times she was outside, at times in the open square,
lurking at every corner.

So she caught him and kissed him;
with an impudent face she said to him:
"I have peace offerings with me;
today I have paid my vows.
So I came out to meet you,
diligently to seek your face,
and I have found you.
I have spread my bed with tapestry,
colored coverings of Egyptian linen.
I have perfumed my bed
with myrrh, aloes, and cinnamon.
Come, let us take our fill of love until morning;
let us delight ourselves with love.
For my husband is not at home;
he has gone on a long journey;
he has taken a bag of money with him,
and will come home on the appointed day."
With her enticing speech she caused him to yield,
with her flattering lips she seduced him.
Immediately he went after her, as an ox goes to the slaughter,
or as a fool to the correction of the stocks,
till an arrow struck his liver.
As a bird hastens to the snare,
he did not know it would cost his life.
Now therefore, listen to me, my children;
pay attention to the words of my mouth:
do not let your heart turn aside to her ways,
do not stray into her paths;
for she has cast down many wounded,
and all who were slain by her were strong men.
Her house is the way to hell,
descending to the chambers of death. (Proverbs 7:6–27)

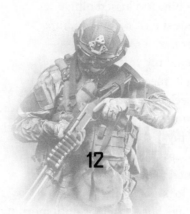

12

FELLOWSHIP

THE SAINT'S WARSHIP

Lay Off the Fluffy Stuff, Bro

Unfortunately, the word *men* and the word *fellowship* seem to clash in the same way that the words *jumbo* and *shrimp* do. Or maybe a peanut butter and sardine sandwich gives a more accurate picture of things that just don't seem to go together very well. This isn't necessarily because men don't like to hang out with other men but mainly because hanging out seems to be the only thing that's on the agenda when bros chill. Opening up and talking about weaknesses, struggles, and sins; digging into the Word together; encouraging one another toward faith and good works; praying with each other—these are just not the sorts of things that men typically do backflips over. In fact, most men would prefer to attempt a neck-breaking backflip or have their toenails ripped out with pliers than to do any of those "fluffy" things with other men. Maybe I'm exaggerating a bit, but two things are certain: (1) It's true that most men don't naturally gravitate toward deep, meaningful engagement with other men, and (2) those things are anything but fluffy.

Flesh-Eating Health

In our quest to be men who walk in (or are controlled by) the Spirit to conquer the lusts of the flesh, we've discussed the fact that we accomplish this by participating in the activities in which the Spirit of God is involved. One of these commonly overlooked and hugely underrated activities is fellowship. In his oft-quoted benediction to God's people, Paul said this to the saints in Corinth: "The grace of the Lord Jesus Christ and the love of God and the fellowship of the Holy Spirit be with you all" (2 Corinthians 13:14 ESV).

When writing to the Philippians, Paul gave this soul-stirring exhortation: "If there is any consolation in Christ, if any comfort of love, if any fellowship of the Spirit, if any affection and mercy, fulfill my joy by being like-minded, having the same love, being of one accord, of one mind" (2:1–2).

The word used here for "fellowship," *koinōnia*, is one of the Greek words from the New Testament that we often hear referenced. Fellowship carries with it the idea of communion, association, intimacy, togetherness, closeness, unity. When the fellowship of the Holy Spirit is "with [us] all" and we are together in fellowship with one another, then there is a special, dynamic connectivity among the Spirit, other believers, and ourselves. Likewise, when the fellowship of the Spirit is in active motion in our lives, then it will result in us being "like-minded" and "having the same love" while "being of one accord" and "of one mind."

The apostle John made a keen connection between the fellowship that believers have with one another and the fellowship that exists between believers and the two other persons of the Trinity who make up the divine Godhead. "That which we have seen and heard we declare to you, that you also may have fellowship with us; and truly our fellowship is with the Father and with His Son Jesus Christ" (1 John 1:3).

A few verses later, John once again showed how the quality of our relationship with God impacts our fellowship with one another as brothers and sisters in Christ: "If we walk in the light as He is in the light, we have fellowship with one another, and the blood of Jesus Christ His Son cleanses us from all sin" (v. 7).

That is one of the sweetest pictures in Scripture of the gospel's outcome in the lives of the redeemed. We walk in the light with God—in all that is pure and righteous and holy—and as we do that, we're drawn into a rich and unifying fellowship with other believers who are walking in that same light. Amid that divine and transformative atmosphere, we, bonded together, experience the benefits of Christ's atoning sacrifice on our behalf—the cleansing effects of His forgiving love.

In the same way that loving God naturally leads to a desire to love our neighbor, so it is that close communion with God leads to a desire to have close communion with other believers. However, don't forget that when we desire to do what is right, we often meet with obstacles and hindrances that seek to derail us in that pursuit. This harkens back to the Galatians 5 Spirit-and-flesh battle that is always raging within us. That's why this Spirit-involved dynamic of fellowship will help us to overcome the flesh.

The Unsinkable Kind of Ship

There are a few common reasons why many Christian men choose to live in isolation. And I'm talking about some men who even have the close fellowship with God that gives them a craving to have fellowship with their Christian brothers. The first reason revolves around a fear of being vulnerable. While the desire to be in close communion with other brothers is there, the fear of appearing weak, sinful, and ungodly overtakes and overwhelms them.

I've often wondered what it would be like if every man were willing to completely let his guard down and open up his life to a small circle of trusted brothers. No holding back, no sugarcoating, no doctoring up their image. Just pure, unadulterated vulnerability, honesty, and candidness. Imagine each man serving his brother with compassion, exhortation, encouragement, prayer, and a challenge to press on in their pursuit of Christ—all the while reminding them of the glorious power found in the precious gospel. If this were to really happen on a grand scale, I believe we would see an unprecedented revival sweep across our planet. It all begins with the realization that God already knows all that there is to know about you as His child and has still accepted you. When you're mindful of this, you'll be more likely to open up your life to other men whom God knows just as intimately and has accepted just as fully as He knows and has accepted you.

This type of fellowship was a major part of the early church's foundation. In fact, it was crucial to their survival amid the hostile atmosphere that they found themselves in as first-century believers. While the winds of persecution were beginning to blow their way, we find that their pursuit of Christ-centered community sustained them and even caused them to richly blossom in the soil of adversity:

> They continued steadfastly in the apostles' doctrine and fellowship, in the breaking of bread, and in prayers. Then fear came upon every soul, and many wonders and signs were done through the apostles. Now all who believed were together, and had all things in common, and sold their possessions and goods, and divided them among all, as anyone had need.
>
> So continuing daily with one accord in the temple, and breaking bread from house to house, they ate their food with gladness and simplicity of heart, praising God and having favor with all the people. And the Lord added to the church daily those who were being saved. (Acts 2:42–47)

Did you notice the distinct attitude with which our faithful predecessors approached their pursuit of fellowship? They did it "steadfastly." This means that they gave unremitting care to it. Thayer's lexicon says that *steadfast* carries the idea of persevering and not fainting in the pursuit of something.[1] Strong's says it means "to be earnest" and "constantly diligent."[2] There was nothing half-hearted or tepid about their endeavor to cultivate dynamic, spiritual synergy with one another. Along with noting their inspirational attitude, we can't help but acknowledge how commendable the components of their fellowship were. We see that they consisted of sitting under the teaching of God's Word ("the apostles' doctrine"), partaking of communion ("the breaking of bread"), and prayer.

---

1   *Thayer's Expanded Greek Definition*, "Proskartereō," StudyLight.org, accessed November 14, 2023, https://www.studylight.org.

2   James Strong, *Strong's Expanded Exhaustive Concordance of the Bible*, Gr. 4342.

While they faced special circumstances that led to the necessity of selling and sharing their goods, we, nonetheless, learn from their spirit of selflessness and generosity. Notice also how this passage in Acts emphasizes community by telling us that "they continued," they "were together," and they were "in one accord."

Plant Them Roots in the Right Soil

All true and fruitful fellowship must have its roots deeply planted in the fertile ground of the local church. In a day and age when individualism is all the rage, when convenience, comfort, and entertainment are huge priorities, faithful membership and proactive involvement in the local church have become optional rather than the nonnegotiable necessities that God has intended them to be.

It is rightly understood that there is no such thing as a church-less Christian. This is because church is not primarily something that Christians participate in; rather, it's something that Christians are. We are the church, His body, the bride of Christ. As such, we should naturally do what the church does—gather together, worship our Redeemer in unity (as we remember His sacrifice and cry out to Him in supplication and praise), and be sharpened by God's Word corporately—all the while selflessly and generously serving and encouraging one another.

And while some may try to justify why they have abandoned gathering with God's people in the context of the local church, there is no justification for it. The misinterpretation of Matthew 18:20—"Where two or three are gathered together in My name, I am there in the midst of them"—and the use of the trite saying "I can worship God anywhere" fly in the face of the norms that the Lord designed, ordained, and established for the functioning of His church.

Hebrews 10 contains the stranded verse that we can use to correct those who discount the importance of Christian fellowship. I'm sure you're familiar with the first part of verse 25: "Not forsaking the assembling of ourselves together, as is the manner of some." While, of course, this is crucial truth, the words that surround that sobering statement, in verse 24 and the rest of verse 25, are crucial for instructing us on why it's important to maintain our togetherness as believers: "Let us consider one another in order to stir up love and good works...exhorting one another, and so much the more as you see the Day approaching."

Stirring up love and good works in one another is a high priority on God's agenda for His people. We're told earlier in Hebrews 11:6 that it's impossible to please God without faith, and the famous verse Romans 1:17 reminds us that "the just shall live by faith." Titus 2:14 says that God wants to "purify for Himself His own special people, zealous for good works," and Ephesians 2:10 makes it clear that we were created in Christ Jesus to do good works.

The author of Hebrews struck a similar tone in verse 13 of chapter 3. He spoke of the importance of exhorting one another every day so that we don't become hardened by the deceitfulness of sin. As nineteenth-century theologian Philip Schaff aptly described, this type of exhortation "includes all the kinds of help, consolation, encouragement, rebuke, which the Christian life needs."[3] Sin is indeed deceitful—seeking to dupe us into forsaking the path of righteousness at every turn. And if we give in to its deceptive lure, we will become hardened under the influence of its corrupting power.

As a man of God who seeks to honor Christ and live a pure and consecrated life, you must make it a nonnegotiable priority to link arms with other men who have the same objective. Men who will not shy away from saying the difficult things that you need to hear, asking the difficult questions that you need to answer, and challenging you to do the difficult things that you need to do. As we've seen, we must begin by doing what the church does and, from there, develop core groups of like-minded men to hold each other accountable.

Godly male friends are more valuable than most men realize, and in his important book *Disciplines of a Godly Man*, R. Kent Hughes effectively highlighted their necessity: "You also need Christian male friends who have a same-sex understanding of the serpentine passages of your heart, who will not only offer counsel and pray for you, but will also hold you accountable to your commitments and responsibilities when necessary."[4]

When speaking of the special bond that Christian men share, Hughes hit it out of the park:

3   Philip Schaff, *A Popular Commentary on the New Testament*, vol. 4 (New York: Charles Scribner's Sons, 1890), 36.
4   R. Kent Hughes, *Disciplines of a Godly Man*, updated ed. (Wheaton, IL: Crossway, 2019), 77.

This is the way it is with deep friendships. It is not that friends think alike on everything. Often it is quite the opposite. But they do share the same worldview and approach to life. And this is why a Christian friendship exceeds anything that exists between nonbelievers—such a friendship is founded on a supernatural mutuality of soul. The Holy Spirit makes two souls chorus the same cries:

- They assent to the same authority.
- They know the same God.
- They go the same way.
- They long for the same things.
- They dream mutual dreams.
- They yearn for the same experiences of holiness and worship.[5]

And then Hughes gave what I believe is one of the most powerful descriptions of what real, God-honoring friendships look like: "The deepest friendships have in common this desire to make the other person royalty. Each works for and rejoices in the other's elevation and achievements. There are no hooks in such friendships, no desire to manipulate or control, no jealousy or exclusiveness—simply a desire for the best for the other. Fyodor Dostoevsky had the idea when he wrote, 'To love a person means to see him as God intended him to be.'"[6]

Teeing Up for Some Real Fellowship

So here are the important elements that must be present for genuine accountability fellowship to thrive and be effective in your life.

Trust

"Things move at the speed of trust" is one of my favorite sayings. Without trust, it's hard to forge ahead effectively and efficiently in any collaborative endeavor. We've all seen the cheesy team-building activities that are designed to develop trust among members of corporate teams. I don't think I can stomach seeing one more person fall back into the arms of their noble coworkers—who heroically catch them and prevent them

---

5   Hughes, *Disciplines of a Godly Man*, 79.
6   Hughes, *Disciplines of a Godly Man*, 81.

from landing on the ground and likely suffering injury. Wow…how very inspiring. How does that ever connect with any type of real-life scenario?

Despite my cynical mockery, the point leaders are trying to convey through such activities (as annoying as they may be) is both admirable and noteworthy. Do you have godly men in your life whom you can safely and confidently depend on? Are they men of character whom you can trust to rebuke you when necessary rather than flatter you with their tongue (Proverbs 28:23)? Are they willing to lovingly wound you for the sake of helping you heal (27:6)? Are you confident that they will regularly pray for you, consistently hold you to account, and lovingly safeguard the sensitive details of your life? It's vital that you find trustworthy men of this ilk and that you demonstrate the same kind of trustworthiness in your life as their friend.

Time

While it's challenging to find trustworthy men with whom to run the race of life, once we have found them, we discover the added challenge of devoting the time necessary to cultivate those crucial relationships and activate the benefits that they produce. Yes, life is busy, energy is limited, and there are only so many hours in a day. However, if we're honest with ourselves, we usually find the time for the things that we really want to do. We somehow make it to the movie theater a couple times a month, watch our favorite sports teams play once or twice a week, or sleep in for two or three extra hours on the weekend. Surely, we can make the time to regularly meet with other Christian men for accountability and fellowship for the sake of our moral purity and spiritual growth. Time invested into these strategic relationships will equal time redeemed for the sake of holiness and the glory of God.

Transparency

Often a direct correlation exists between how transparent we choose to be and how much our accountability with other men helps us. As I've already mentioned, we typically try to hide who we really are or doctor up our image because we're worried about what others might think about us if they discover how sinful we really are. But as Paul David Tripp so aptly put it, "When you live out of the grace of the gospel, you quit fearing failure, you quit avoiding being known, and you quit hiding your struggles and your sin. The gospel declares that there is nothing that could ever be uncovered about you and me that hasn't already been covered by the grace of Jesus."[7]

You have to cling to the fact that God knows your sinfulness better than anyone else ever could, and He demonstrated His love toward you by sending Jesus to die for you while you were still a sinner (Romans 5:8). Let this knowledge fill you with a sense of security and then move you to be completely open with your brothers about your specific sins and struggles—both past and present. Remember, you're not confessing your sins to your trusted friends so that you can receive forgiveness from them. That happens between you and the Lord because "in Him we have redemption through His blood, the forgiveness of sins" (Ephesians 1:7). You're doing it so that they can exhort you, encourage you, remind you of truth, and, most importantly, pray for you (James 5:16).

As Heath Lambert reminded us, "We are not designed to pull our way out of our spiritual ruts in our own strength. We need the help of other Christians. You will never be free from pornography until you acknowledge that in order to change you need the help of God through brothers…in Christ."[8]

When you choose to become completely transparent with the men who are a part of your accountability fellowship group, your example will often compel them to be completely transparent as well. And from there, wonderful things begin to happen.

Teachability

Having counseled many people over the course of my nearly thirty years in ministry, I've often had to ask God for help when I hear the same recurring response from people I advise. To my chagrin, I've allowed it to become a pet peeve at times, and I really wish it weren't. Perhaps you've also experienced it. Someone comes to you for advice, so you lovingly pour out your heart and share with them as much truth as you can from God's Word. However, every time you dispense some bit of advice,

---

7   Paul David Tripp, *Dangerous Calling: Confronting the Unique Challenges of Pastoral Ministry* (Wheaton, IL: Crossway, 2015), 99.
8   Heath Lambert, *Finally Free: Fighting for Purity with the Power of Grace* (Grand Rapids, MI: Zondervan, 2013), 46.

they respond by saying, "I know." And it's not the agreeable type of "I know," as in, "Oh, yeah, wow—I know," meant to convey that they're fully tracking with you and are totally in harmony with what you're saying. It's more of the know-it-all type of "I know" with a splash of attitude.

We do both ourselves and our friends a huge disservice when we don't have a teachable spirit. We miss out on gaining helpful input that could greatly impact our lives, and they miss out on experiencing the joy of sensing that the Lord has genuinely used them to help us. The last thing you want is for your friends to hold back on speaking into your life because your attitude gives them the impression that you can't gain anything beneficial from them. And if you flat out hate receiving correction, then you're just plain stupid. Yes, if that's you, I did just call you that—but our Father did it first: "Whoever loves instruction loves knowledge, but he who hates correction is stupid" (Proverbs 12:1).

The good news is that there's hope for the stupid (and which of us hasn't been stupid at some point). We can learn to become lovers of correction and counsel and instruction, and by God's grace, we can turn from stupid to wise: "Listen to counsel and receive instruction, that you may be wise in your latter days" (Proverbs 19:20).

Time, trust, transparency, and teachability—these are the necessary components for healthy accountability fellowship, which is the natural fruit produced from first thriving in the nutrient-rich soil of the local church. And this will become the healthy catalyst that will unleash into your life the transformative power that comes from really living in genuine biblical community—the type of transformative power that will help to kill lustful desires in your heart and fuel purity in the very core of your being.

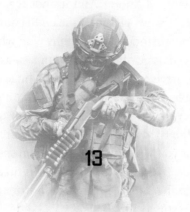

13

EVANGELISM

THE DISCIPLE'S SECRET WEAPON

Power Surge

After Jesus died and rose again and just before He ascended to the Father, He said something of massive significance to His disciples: "You shall receive power when the Holy Spirit has come upon you; and you shall be witnesses to Me in Jerusalem, and in all Judea and Samaria, and to the end of the earth" (Acts 1:8).

Evangelism, therefore, is the fourth and final element in which God's Spirit is directly involved.

Bet You Didn't See That Coming

One of the staff members who serves at our ministry told us a gripping story about his brother who was living in Utah several years ago. One day a group of masked men took the man's brother and pushed him into the back room of a building. They knocked him out, cut his chest open with a knife, and ripped out his heart. And what's more is that there were people outside that room who knew what was going on and had the power to stop it, but they were unwilling to intervene.

Now let me give you some more information. That group of masked men were heart surgeons. Their knives were scalpels. They pushed the man on a gurney. The back room of that building was the operating room of a hospital. They knocked him out with anesthesia, they cut his chest open surgically, and they removed his heart because it was damaged and needed to be replaced with a good one. And no one did anything to stop it because they cared about the man and wanted him to get better.

You just experienced a very powerful dynamic called a *paradigm shift*. A paradigm shift occurs when you have a particular perspective on something, and then you receive new bits of information that radically alter your perspective. What you were sure was a gruesome murder scene instantly transformed into a life-saving operation.

Let me present to you a different paradigm shift. Let's start with a passage of Scripture that sheds light on some of the spiritual gifts that God sovereignly dispenses to select individuals within His kingdom: "He Himself gave some to be apostles, some prophets, some evangelists, and some pastors and teachers" (Ephesians 4:11).

Perhaps as you read this list, you logically conclude that God has not gifted you in any of those select areas. You, therefore, reason that you're not required to do any of the things that are related to those specific realms of ministry. I would venture to guess that the activities you're most relieved about not having to participate in are the ones directly related to the evangelist. The thought of talking to friends, family members, and strangers about the state of their eternal souls is enough to send you into a full-blown panic attack. So I'm sure you're wiping the sweat off your brow right about now.

However, maybe a little more information will be the inspiration that will cause you more perspiration. We find that information in the very next verse, where we read that Jesus gave these gifts "for the equipping of the saints for the work of ministry, for the edifying of the body of Christ" (v. 12). This sure puts a whole different spin on things, doesn't it? While the evangelist most certainly evangelizes, Paul told us in our text that one of the evangelist's primary roles is to equip the saints for the work of ministry. God has uniquely gifted evangelists to disciple disciples in the ministry of disciple making.

So what exactly does this all mean for you? It means that God has given you a divine calling to proclaim the precious gospel of Christ to a lost and dying world. Is this not the mandate that Jesus gave to the apostles and that they, in turn, passed on to us as members of the body of Christ?

Here is that Great Commission that has led to the transformation of the world and that ultimately resulted in your own conversion: "Jesus came and spoke to them, saying, 'All authority has been given to Me in heaven and on earth. Go therefore and make disciples of all the nations, baptizing them in the name of the Father and of the Son and of the Holy Spirit, teaching them to observe all things that I have commanded you; and lo, I am with you always, even to the end of the age.' Amen" (Matthew 28:18–20). Additionally, Paul said in 2 Corinthians 5:18–20 that all believers have been given the ministry of reconciliation and are called to be ambassadors for Christ.

Perhaps this comes as a shock to you, but you are currently in full-time ministry. You may be thinking that pastors, missionaries, and Christian counselors are the only kinds of people who are in full-time ministry. However, if you are a Christian who has been reconciled to Christ, then God has called you to be a minister of the same reconciliation you've received, and He has given you the official role and title of ambassador for Christ.

You may be thinking, *Wait a minute. I didn't sign up for this. I'm not really interested in that sort of ministry, role, or title.* Oh well; that's really too bad. This is an indisputable reality that has nothing to do with your preferences or desires. If you have been born again, you are as much a minister of reconciliation and an ambassador for Christ as you are a human being if you've been born to a human father and mother. It may not be surprising these days that there are some people who prefer to identify as something other than human, but while they can pretend all they want, facts are stubborn things that don't yield or bow to delusional fantasies.

People don't often ask if a man or a woman is a human being, but on the basis of how someone lives their life, people might rightly ask a person, *What kind of human being are you?* There are faithful human beings and unfaithful human beings, responsible human beings and irresponsible human beings, committed human beings and uncommitted human beings. And the same holds true for every Christian.

So here's the paradigm shift: if you are truly a child of the living God, then you are a full-time minister of reconciliation and an ambassador for Christ. That's irrefutable. The real question is, What kind of minister and ambassador are you?

Poised to Passionately Please

Earlier on in 2 Corinthians 5, Paul began building a case that lays the foundation for our calling to live as ambassadors for Christ and ministers of reconciliation: "We make it our aim, whether present or absent, to be well pleasing to Him. For we must all appear before the judgment seat of Christ, that each one may receive the things done in the body, according to what he has done, whether good or bad" (2 Corinthians 5:9–10).

Paul was saying that it should be the Christian's aim and ambition in life, whether they are in time or in eternity, to be well pleasing to God. In keeping with this noble goal, I gathered my wife and kids in our living room many years ago and unveiled for them a special vision statement that I had crafted for our family. It reads like this: "To gladly and passionately glorify God in every thought, affection, word, and deed while constantly enjoying Him as our greatest pleasure and most precious treasure."

Along with emblazoning this family vision statement on a large plaque that hangs on our living room wall, I've memorized it, my wife has memorized it, and each one of our five children has memorized it. It has become a regular topic of discussion in our home and a popular theme for our family devotions. Because if there is anything that I want my children to know—and their children to know—it's that they were made by God and for God and that their ambition should be to glorify Him in everything they think, feel, say, and do as they live to bring Him pleasure and enjoy Him across the entire spectrum of their lives (as the first question and answer of the Westminster Shorter Catechism states).

In connection with this, Paul reminded us that there is coming a day when we are going to stand before the judgment seat of Christ and give an account of the way we lived. Did we truly live to please God, or did we live for our own agenda and self-gratification? While this is not the great white throne judgment mentioned in Scripture (Revelation 20:11–15), from which God will condemn those who refused to repent and place their faith in Christ, this will nonetheless be a time of serious reckoning for believers.

This judgment seat of Christ (previously highlighted in chapter 7 of this book) is called the *bema* seat in the original Greek language. It's been compared to the seat on which an athletics judge would sit at the end of a particular competition during ancient games and from which he would dispense rewards to those who competed faithfully and successfully. If we do not wholeheartedly run the race that God has marked out for us, the tragedy is that we will have failed to maximize our full capacity to glorify the Lord and will end up forfeiting wonderful eternal rewards that could have been ours. We don't know exactly what those rewards are, but whatever comes from the hand of God is perfect and something we should always desire.

Some have conjectured that the rewards will come in the form of our capacity to enjoy God or shine for His glory in eternity. While all of us will enjoy God and shine for His glory to the fullness of our capacity, the capacity of each person's fullness may vary depending on the degree of their surrender and obedience to the Lord in every area of life. Some of us may have the capacity of an Olympic-size swimming pool, while others might have the capacity of a bathtub. Again, those capacities will be filled to the brim with the fullness of the enjoyment of God and the privilege of shining for His glory, and we may not personally notice any difference, but we may end up receiving much less than what we could have. Again, no one is certain about this as the Bible is not clear on it, but it's definitely worth contemplating.

Paul touched on the whole concept of receiving and losing rewards in 1 Corinthians:

> According to the grace of God which was given to me, as a wise master builder I have laid the foundation, and another builds on it. But let each one take heed how he builds on it. For no other foundation can anyone lay than that which is laid, which is Jesus Christ. Now if anyone builds on this foundation with gold, silver, precious stones, wood, hay,

straw, each one's work will become clear; for the Day will declare it, because it will be revealed by fire; and the fire will test each one's work, of what sort it is. If anyone's work which he has built on it endures, he will receive a reward. If anyone's work is burned, he will suffer loss; but he himself will be saved, yet so as through fire. (3:10–15)

In light of how short time is and how long eternity will be, how passionate should we be about no longer living to please ourselves but instead living to wholeheartedly please the Lord? I realize this will be difficult for you to believe, but shortly before his recent passing, we celebrated my father's one hundred thirteenth birthday. Even though he was sixty-five when I was born, yes, he was my biological father (who married my much younger mother). I know that one hundred thirteen years may seem like a very long time, and relatively speaking, it is. However, it's not even a blip in comparison to eternity.

James reminds us that our life is but a vapor. It's like hot breath on cold air. It appears for a brief second and then quickly vanishes. I assure you that, to my dad, his one hundred thirteen years passed by quicker than the blink of an eye. Let's not waste the time God has given us; let's invest it in eternal causes as we live for the pleasure of God.

The John 3:16 Syndrome

This calling to invest our lives in living for God's pleasure is not baseless; it has its roots in something that Paul said in 2 Corinthians: "He died for all, that those who live should live no longer for themselves, but for Him who died for them and rose again" (5:15).

How do the words of that verse strike you? As a longtime student of the Bible, I've often felt convicted by how desensitized I sometimes become to certain truths in God's Word. It's almost like I allow particular portions of Scripture to become overfamiliar to me. That sounds ridiculous! How is that even possible? You would think that the more intimately acquainted we become with what the Lord has revealed, the more those truths will grip us. This should certainly be the case, and in many instances, it is. But if we aren't careful and intentional, we can begin to take truth—even extremely powerful truth—for granted. I call it

the John 3:16 Syndrome. Most Christians can rattle that verse off in their
sleep, maybe even backward. However, because we've had it memorized
for so long or have heard it so often, sometimes our hearts don't connect
with its significance.

So with that in mind, read those words from 2 Corinthians again:
"He died for all, that those who live should live no longer for themselves,
but for Him who died for them and rose again."

Did you catch that? Christ died! The pure, holy, spotless, righteous, exalted, eternal Son of God—God the Son, the second person of
the triune Godhead—died. He left the splendors of heaven and robed
Himself in human flesh. He endured the blasphemies that came from the
lips, tongues, and vocal cords He fashioned. He was nailed to a rugged
piece of wood that came from a tree that He created. He was pierced with
spikes that were formed from earthly elements that He produced. And
then, He died.

How much do you value the fact that Christ died for you, Christian?

In his powerful book *Dangerous Calling*, Paul David Tripp masterfully demonstrated how the things we value affect our behavior. I'd like to
briefly highlight his important insights and expand on them a bit.

Dr. Tripp gave a powerful illustration about a twenty-dollar bill
and how its value is not intrinsic. In other words, the bill is not worth
twenty dollars because of the paper it's printed on or because of the ink
on the paper. Otherwise, you'd need a huge stack of paper and a bucket
full of ink in order to match that value. No, the note is worth twenty dollars because the US government has assigned that value to it. Because we
acknowledge the US government as an official authority, that assigned
value then influences how we behave toward the twenty-dollar bill.
Likewise, the government has assigned to that other round, copper piece
of currency that often jangles annoyingly in our pockets a value that is a
mere two-thousandth of that twenty-dollar bill.

Our knowledge of that assigned value is the reason why we sometimes don't bother to stoop down and pick up a penny when we pass by
one lying somewhere on the ground. But we would never behave that
way toward a twenty-dollar bill, would we? However, imagine if the US
government decided to switch those values, and suddenly the penny
became worth twenty dollars and the twenty-dollar bill became worth a

penny. You can be sure that your behavior would change because of those switched values. First, you'd weep buckets of tears over all the pennies you didn't pick up and save because you would have probably become a millionaire, and then you'd begin using the twenty-dollar bills as pieces of scrap paper or napkins to wipe your hands with.[1]

So let me ask you again: How much do you value the sacrificial death of Christ on your behalf? Had God the Father not willed to assign a redemptive value to the crucifixion of Christ, then it would provide no salvific benefits to you whatsoever. But God the Father has most certainly assigned that redemptive value to Christ's substitutionary atonement on behalf of sinners. Do you acknowledge the Father's supreme and official authority, and do you, therefore, value the fact that Christ died? If you do, then your behavior should be radically impacted by that reality. It should translate into you no longer living for yourself but for Him who died for you and rose again.

Newer Than New Car Smell

As Paul continued to construct his powerful argument, he laid one more important brick. He said something in verse 17 that is no doubt quite familiar to most Christians: "If anyone is in Christ, he is a new creation; old things have passed away; behold, all things have become new" (2 Corinthians 5:17).

We often quote this verse in isolation, and it's not uncommon to see it painted or printed on Christian artwork and hanging in churches or homes. But in context, it directly relates to the Christian's death to self and his abandonment of living for his own pleasure. As a new creation, you have done away with those old selfish things, and as a believer, you should now walk in the newness of living to please the God who gave His life to save you.

Cook My Own What?

We've seen how Paul has informed us in 2 Corinthians 5 of several important truths:

---

1   Paul David Tripp, *Dangerous Calling: Confronting the Unique Challenges of Pastoral Ministry* (Wheaton, IL: Crossway, 2015), 102–4.

1. This life that we are to live should have the aim of pleasing God as its sole ambition.
2. We will one day stand before the judgment seat of Christ and give an account for how we lived.
3. Christ died and rose again so that we would no longer live for our own pleasures but for His.
4. This is all possible because the things associated with our old, selfish life of living for ourselves and our own pleasures have passed away, and all things, through our regeneration, have become new.

Having communicated these things, the apostle crescendoed with the verses that I first highlighted when we began our exploration of this passage in 2 Corinthians:

> All things are of God, who has reconciled us to Himself through Jesus Christ, and has given us the ministry of reconciliation, that is, that God was in Christ reconciling the world to Himself, not imputing their trespasses to them, and has committed to us the word of reconciliation.
>
> Now then, we are ambassadors for Christ, as though God were pleading through us: we implore you on Christ's behalf, be reconciled to God. (5:18–20)

With the full context now in mind, hopefully you're beginning to experience the significant aspects of this revolutionary paradigm shift. However, it's also possible for you to be feeling quite overwhelmed at this point. It's extremely daunting to be given the responsibilities associated with being an ambassador for Christ and a minister of reconciliation. But I want you to be encouraged by the fact that if God has called you to do something, He will most certainly give you everything you will need to accomplish it. Is this not what a nation does when it sends ambassadors to another country? All that nation's resources will be at those ambassadors' disposal as they go about the task of representing their homeland.

Ephesians 2:10 gives us a glimpse into this blessed provision: "We are His workmanship, created in Christ Jesus for good works, which God prepared beforehand that we should walk in them."

EVANGELISM

Prepared is one of my favorite words in the English language. It's all the more delightful to me when it's coupled with the word *beforehand*, especially when those two words are used in connection with the word *food*.

I grew up in a Middle Eastern home, and if you know anything about Middle Eastern mothers, you understand that they are quite famous for spoiling their kids rotten—especially their sons. My mom began to clue in on the fact that her attempts to lovingly nurture me were actually beginning to handicap me. So one day, when I asked her to make me a sandwich, which was normal protocol, she gave me an earful. She told me that I needed to learn to make my own sandwiches because she feared I would inevitably marry a woman who would never take care of me and feed me the way that she did, and I would, therefore, end up starving. My mom was right about a lot of things, but she was definitely wrong about that. My wonderful wife, Rachel, has kept this helpless man alive, and she very kindly prepares my food beforehand—well, at least most of the time. In honor of my beautiful late mother's memory, I've become quite an accomplished sandwich-making connoisseur.

Many years ago, some friends of ours told us about a restaurant called the Melting Pot that served the most amazing chocolate fondue. They talked about how chocolate chunks melt in a bowl that sits on a burner affixed to your table. They mesmerized me with descriptions of dipping marshmallows, bananas, strawberries, and graham crackers into the fondue. Being a raging chocoholic, I couldn't make reservations at the restaurant fast enough. After we arrived and ordered our fondue and dinner, I could hardly hear a word that my beloved wife said as we waited. I couldn't care less about the dinner because I was transfixed on that chocolaty taste of heaven that I was sure would change my life forever.

Before long, our server approached our table with bowls of raw meat, raw chicken, and raw vegetables. I was completely puzzled. By the look on the server's face, after he saw the look on my face, I could tell that he had seen that same look on many other men's faces. "Oh, yes, you actually cook your own food here," he said. *Wait, wait, wait! He said what? I do what to my own what here?* I thought the whole point of going to a restaurant is *not* to have to cook your own food. Did these preeminent masters of all things chocolaty forget that the first part of the word *restaurant* is *rest*? I could imagine the diabolical genius who hatched this evil scheme rubbing his hands together in the kitchen and saying, "Lure them here, make them cook their own food, and charge them twice the going rate. Bwahahahaha!"

When we finished eating, I half expected someone to escort us to the back to wash our own dishes.

Unlike the shrewd people at that restaurant, God doesn't do this to His people. He doesn't call us to the most important task in the universe—representing Him as His ambassadors through the ministry of reconciliation—and then tell us to figure out how to do it on our own. As we just saw, He has actually prepared beforehand all our good works (which include evangelistic good works) that we should walk in them.

I Want to Be a Golden Goblet

Here comes paradigm shift number two: "In a great house there are not only vessels of gold and silver, but also of wood and clay, some for honor and some for dishonor. Therefore, if anyone cleanses himself from the latter, he will be a vessel for honor, sanctified and useful for the Master, prepared for every good work" (2 Timothy 2:20–21).

Paul told us in Ephesians that our evangelistic good works are prepared beforehand for us, and now his words tell us in 2 Timothy that we can be prepared for every one of those good works. In context, we do this by "cleansing ourselves from the latter," which means putting off a dishonorable life and walking uprightly with the Lord as vessels of honor.

This means that as we regularly walk along the path of life as ambassadors for Christ who are fulfilling our ministry of reconciliation, there are these amazing, prepackaged good works of evangelism, like giant gift-wrapped boxes that God has meticulously prepared for us beforehand. And as we conduct ourselves in holiness, we are, in turn, prepared for these good works. What happens is that we and these good works of evangelism, both being prepared for one another, end up providentially intersecting at perfect points in time and space in what I call divine convergences.

It's Wonderful to Feel Used

If you've never had the pleasure of experiencing a divine convergence, you know that it's one of the most extraordinary privileges in existence.

Before I came to know Christ, one of the things I despised most was the sense that I had been used by someone. And anytime I heard a friend say that another person used them, I always knew that very negative details were about to follow. But as Christians, is there any greater honor than for us to be able to say that we were used by God? And especially when He uses us as instruments to bring the gospel of light and life to lost and hopeless souls.

Sometimes we're not struck with the appropriate measure of awe and sobriety when it comes to our calling as ambassadors for Christ whom He has entrusted with the ministry of reconciliation. This is often the case because we make too much of ourselves and too little of God. We forget who He really is and who we are in comparison to Him.

I love this powerful contrast that I heard a pastor share many years ago. If we were to hop on a beam of light and fly through space at the speed of light, 186,000 miles per second, it would take us about a second and a half to reach the moon. In about eight minutes, we'd be at the sun, ninety-three million miles away. In four years, we would collide with Alpha Centauri, the closest star system to our own solar system. But if we started our trek at the beginning of our galaxy, the Milky Way, and traveled all the way across it to the other end, it would take us one hundred thousand years to complete our journey. There are between one hundred and two hundred billion galaxies in the universe with trillions of stars sprinkled across those galaxies, and the Bible tells us that our God measures the universe with His hand (Isaiah 40:12) and that heaven and the heaven of heavens can't contain Him (2 Chronicles 2:6). So in reality, we are specks of dust upon a speck of dust, floating through a speck of dust, within a speck of dust, and the infinite God, who became a speck of dust in order to redeem us, has called us to be His representatives. Is this radical reality not enough to rouse us out of our slumber, to enlighten us to the privilege we've been given, and to enthuse us to take seriously the sacred calling with which we've been entrusted?

The Beatles Fan and the Fearful Flyer

I'd like to whet your appetite for evangelism and inspire you to begin embarking on evangelistic adventures of your own by sharing a few divine convergences from my life. Over the course of more than twenty-five years, I've had the opportunity to travel quite a bit as a pastor and as the president of Living Waters ministry. That being the case, one of my favorite places to carry out my ministry of reconciliation as an ambassador for Christ is on airplanes. As Ray Comfort often says, if you're sharing the gospel with someone when you're thirty thousand feet in the air and they don't like it, you can simply say, "There's the door."

A few years ago, Ray and I were flying back home from an out-of-state speaking trip. After boarding the plane, I sat down next to a young man in his early twenties who looked quite friendly. After striking up a conversation with him and talking about a variety of things, I ended up making a natural transition into sharing my testimony and then the gospel. My new friend responded with respect and openness. I then reached into my backpack to pull out a DVD of a movie our ministry had produced called *Audacity*. I thought it would be the perfect fit for him.

However, as I pulled the DVD out, I realized that I had grabbed the wrong one. I had forgotten that I had also brought DVDs of another movie we had released called *Genius* about the life of John Lennon, one of the Beatles. The movie starts out exploring Lennon's life and then segues into the gospel. Having already pulled out the wrong movie but thinking that it was a long shot that this young man was even familiar with the Beatles, I hesitantly asked him anyway if he had ever heard of them. To my utter surprise, his eyes got as wide as saucers, and he excitedly exclaimed, "I'm a huge Beatles fan—no, I'm an insane Beatles fan!" I replied, "Hey, man! Let it be. All you need is love right now." No, I didn't really say that, but I wish I had.

In the meantime, a few rows in front of me, Ray Comfort sat next to a young lady who was serving in the US Air Force and who also happened to be deathly afraid of flying. Yes, like you, I was also scratching my head over that one. Some people need a ray of hope, but this lady needed a Ray of Comfort, and she certainly got one. After consoling her and putting her mind at ease about the flight, Ray discovered that she had Jewish roots. Being of Jewish descent himself, he proceeded to share the gospel with her, telling her about Jesus, the Jewish Messiah. At the end of the conversation, he asked her if she believed that Jesus is the Messiah. She looked at him and said, "Now I do."

After walking off the plane and excitedly exchanging stories with Ray, I had a nagging sense that something wasn't right. I pulled out my phone and checked our flight itinerary to look at our assigned seating arrangements. Sure enough, Ray and I were originally given seats 20A and 20B. However, because we checked in separately at different kiosks, our seats were changed. I "just happened" to get placed next to a mega Beatles fan and equipped with a DVD about the Beatles, and Ray, the Jew, "coincidentally" ended up next to a gal of Jewish heritage who was afraid of flying and needed comfort—along with an introduction to the Jewish Messiah. Divine convergence!

Arabs like Cherubs in the Sky

On another homebound journey, it looked like I was going to get some extra elbow room. As I sat next to the window, I was delighted to see that there was an open spot between the passenger who was sitting in the aisle seat and me. Now this is always a welcomed treat for those who do a lot of traveling. Having a little added space to stretch out a bit can make all the difference on a long flight.

After they announced that the door had been closed, I was certain that my heart's desire had been granted. But just as I was about to spread out and get comfortable, I noticed one more passenger making his way down the aisle. And here's where my flesh and spirit launched World War III against one another. My spirit was hoping he was sitting next to me so that I could share the gospel with him, but my weary flesh was really hoping that this ambassador for Christ could have a day off. As the young man got closer and closer to my row, I began to resign myself to the fact that it was looking like the Lord was calling me to report for duty after all. Sure enough, before I knew it, my new traveling companion plopped down next to me, and my heart shifted from selfish murmuring to gratitude and prayer.

From the moment that I greeted the fine gentleman who would be my neighbor for a few hours, I could tell that we were going to really get along. We hit it off rather quickly, and I was very impressed with how intelligent, well-spoken, and witty he was. At one point in the course of our stimulating conversation, I asked him if he lived in the state where we had boarded our plane or if he was from California, the state where

I live and to which we were headed. To my utter shock, he responded by saying, "Oh, I've never been to America before. I just got here a few hours ago."

I was quite befuddled by this. The guy spoke almost perfect English; I could hardly even detect an accent. "Where are you from?" I asked in complete bewilderment.

I nearly fell out of my seat when he looked at me and said, "Lebanon."

Huh? It took a second for my brain to process that. So then I blurted out, "*Marhaba*," which is the Arabic word for "hello." He looked at me and calmly replied, "Oh, that's pretty good."

I said, "No, man. I'm Lebanese!" I then unleashed a barrage of Arabic on him.

Now he was the one who was stunned. We both sat there in disbelief for a second and then started chatting like two long-lost friends. As our conversation progressed, I eventually began witnessing to him. I found out that he had a Muslim background but didn't consider himself to be a very religious person. He seemed extremely engaged in our conversation and was both courteous and interactive. It turned out that he was a college student who was headed to Orange County for a summer study abroad program at a university. As our plane was about to land, my friend seemed a bit disconcerted. He told me that he wasn't sure what to do because he may have arrived a day too early and the school might not be ready to accommodate him in his dorm room. However, his phone was not operational in the United States yet, and he didn't know how he would even contact the school. Of course, I told him he could use my phone once we debarked our plane.

Sure enough, after he called the school, my new friend confirmed that he had indeed arrived a day too early. He had no place to stay for the night, he had no mode of transportation, his phone wasn't operational, and he didn't know a soul in California.

Well, now he did. It just so happened that this was one of the first times I had parked my car at the airport. I would typically have someone drop me off and pick me up. But God orchestrated things for His sovereign purposes on this day. I joyfully looked over at my friend and told him not to worry about a thing. We hopped in my car and hit the road.

He had told me on the plane that he was a sushi fanatic (like me), so off we went, and I treated him to a delicious sushi dinner. After finishing our meal, I drove him over to a local hotel, booked a room for him, and paid for it. I could see the wonder in his eyes and sensed in him the recognition that none of the things that happened were coincidental.

I'm happy to say that the two of us have maintained a connection through the years. I was so delighted when he wrote to me and pointed out his amazement over how he ended up next to me—the Lebanese guy—out of the hundreds of seats that were on that plane. And my heart melted when he spoke about how touched his parents were by the way one of their fellow countrymen had taken care of their son while he was in a foreign land on the other side of the planet. Divine convergence!

A Cop Who Gave Away Millions

Whenever I travel, I typically like to take one of my five children with me. Some time ago, I was invited to speak at a conference in Ohio, and I took along my then thirteen-year-old son Luke on that trip. In the course of our journey, we found ourselves traveling through one of the busiest airports in the United States of America. After making it through security, which is often a miracle for this very innocent-looking Arab, Luke pointed to the left and said, "Dad, look, isn't that one of Living Waters' *Million Dollar Bill* gospel tracts?" I looked to my left and saw a counter with three police officers behind it and a rectangular object sitting on a little stand. After walking over to the counter, I immediately noticed that my son was wrong. It was not one of my ministry's *Million Dollar Bill* gospel tracts; it was an entire stack of them!

At this point, one of the police officers began walking toward me. As I stood there in a *The Twilight Zone* sort of daze, I opened my mouth and said, "Excuse me, sir. My ministry prints these tracts, and I have no idea how they got here."

He then looked at me and exclaimed, "E.Z.!" It felt like it was some sort of sting operation, and I almost yelled out, *I had nothing to do with this! It's Ray Comfort's fault!* He went on to tell me about how much he loved Living Waters and what we do.

Then it suddenly dawned on me, and I asked, "Sir, did you put these tracts here?" He enthusiastically informed me that he had. I then asked, "And they haven't stopped you yet?" I remember wondering how it was that this brother hadn't gotten busted.

He shot back at me with a big smile and a hearty, "Not yet!"

I was so blown away by all this that I gave the officer my card and asked him to email me. I was very eager to hear the backstory behind this unusual turn of events. When I got back home from my trip to Ohio, I found the following email from the officer in my inbox:

> Good morning, sir,
>
> As the subject line says, it was nice to meet you and your son yesterday at [the airport].
>
> Yesterday was the first time I have ever set the tracts out at the law enforcement podium, even though the thought occurred to me a few years ago when I first learned of your ministry through a homeschool conference…
>
> When my two partners and I arrived at the podium yesterday, I pulled out the tracts to set them up. They were curious and read the tract, including the gospel message on the back. That then sparked a conversation that lasted several hours.
>
> I used info from Ray Comfort, Voddie Baucham, Ken Ham, and all the other info I've picked up from a variety of sources, like the Bible. They weren't getting it. They challenged me on everything from ancient aliens to why Jews are God's chosen people.
>
> Then you walked up. After you left, I had to explain who you were and the total improbability of you walking up at that moment. As one of my partners put it, it was like having an Amazon Kindle on display, talking about Amazon products, and then Jeff Bezos walking up.
>
> Using God's blessing of mobile internet, I showed them LivingWaters.com, *180*, *Noah*, *Evolution vs. God*, and whatever else was up on the screen. After a ten-hour shift of witnessing, I believe they will begin following Christ.[2]

---

2 Email communication was slightly edited for readability and clarity.

I'm sure you can imagine the bliss that shot through my body when I read that email. This was one of the highlights of my life as a Christian. As the officer himself said, and as one of his partners affirmed, think of the "total improbability" of something like that happening by chance. Of all the days I could have been traveling, it was that day; of all the multiple airports we could have traveled through, it was that airport; of all the many security checkpoints we could have entered at that airport, it was that particular one; of all the different directions in which my son could have looked after we cleared security, it was in that direction; of all the hundreds of days that the officer had considered putting the tracts on the podium—over the course of "a few years"—that was the specific day he chose; and of all the things he could have been doing at the very moment that I walked up, he was sharing the gospel from my ministry's gospel tract. Those who don't believe in the existence of God really have problems! Divine convergence!

High-Octane Motivation

As I mentioned before I started sharing those stories and as you saw in each one of them, my good works of evangelism were prepared beforehand, and I was prepared for my good works of evangelism. God then caused them to intersect at a perfect point in time and space in splendid divine convergences. To Him be the glory!

I hope that your heart was as stirred by reading about those amazing encounters as mine was while experiencing them and recounting them to you. It's difficult for a believer who walks in the Spirit by regularly sharing his faith to easily give in to sexual temptations. This is because the consciousness of the gospel's power and God's ability to transform and liberate from sin are ever before his eyes. And the desire to continue to be used by God in something as important as delivering a message through which the Lord can save people from eternal damnation and give them the gift of everlasting life is an ongoing and massive motivation. Not to mention the distaste he will develop at the thought of walking in hypocrisy by living in sexual immorality while constantly preaching to others that they should repent of the very same sin.

When This Exceeds That, Then This, That, and the Other Happen

Now I realize that fear is often the paralyzing element that keeps many of us from sharing the gospel. I want you to know that you're not alone in this regard. I'm the president of a ministry that mainly focuses on winning souls and training others to do the same. I've shared the gospel all over the world with more people than I can count. However, I still deal with fear at times. And believe it or not, so does Ray Comfort. He's been proclaiming the gospel since the early 1970s, and he began by open-air preaching almost every weekday for twelve years in New Zealand. But as the saying goes, "Courage is not the absence of fear. It's the conquering of it."

Many years ago, when Ray and I were speaking at an evangelism training conference in New Zealand, I was greatly impacted by a slogan that the organizers had printed on T-shirts for participants: "When desperation exceeds our fears, progress begins." How so very true that is. And you can fill that blank in with so many different legitimate things. When care, concern, sympathy, love, and compassion exceed our fears, progress begins. Something far more important must outweigh the fears that are holding us back in order for us to realize evangelistic progress.

One of the biggest killers of evangelistic zeal is concern over what people might think of us. When I was a very young man, I started an evangelism team through the church that I had co-planted. When I took our group out on the streets for the first time, I was absolutely terrified. But then a thought entered my mind that really helped calm my heart and propel me to open my mouth in love. It was simply this: *Stop caring about what people think and begin to think about caring for people.* It was really eye-opening for me. I realized that I cared so much about what people thought of me that I didn't pause long enough to think about caring for people—whose eternal destiny was the lake of fire if they didn't repent and place their faith in Christ. As my focus shifted and I started to gear my heart and mind in this new direction, my attitude changed, and that led to the transformation of my conduct. I began pushing myself beyond the boundaries of my comfort zone, casting aside my apprehensions, and doing what I knew was right despite what I felt.

Say Amen or Ouch

Ray Comfort often issues a challenge that is perhaps the most convicting I've ever heard. He asks people if they would be willing to set aside their fears and share the gospel with others if they received $10,000 each time they did it within the course of one twenty-four-hour period. He insists that this would lead to 4 a.m. evangelism outreaches around the world. The alarm clock that people so hate would suddenly become their best friend when it rings at that early, forbidding hour. They would grab a flashlight, a pen and pad, and a calculator and practically knock down people's doors and drag them out of bed so that they could tell them about Christ. And then, Ray hits everyone with the big kicker: "Are you willing to deal with your fear of man problem out of your love for money and not out of your love for God?" As one famous preacher so aptly put it, "If you can't say amen, you ought to say ouch."[3]

A Symphony of Sympathy

It's crucial that this chapter ends on a very high note of encouragement. It's most definitely not the Lord's desire for you to walk away discouraged over such an important and wonderful topic. You must know God's heart toward you amid your battle with fear, failure, indifference, and discouragement when it comes to engaging in the Spirit-driven activity of evangelism.

Here is what Scripture declares loudly and clearly to you: "Seeing then that we have a great High Priest who has passed through the heavens, Jesus the Son of God, let us hold fast our confession. For we do not have a High Priest who cannot sympathize with our weaknesses, but was in all points tempted as we are, yet without sin. Let us therefore come boldly to the throne of grace, that we may obtain mercy and find grace to help in time of need" (Hebrews 4:14–16).

Is that not absolutely mind-blowing? The God of the universe is telling you that He was tempted with every external, general temptation that has ever tempted you. There is nothing you've ever encountered in that regard that He Himself doesn't understand. While, of course, He never gave in to those temptations, He nevertheless experienced them.

3   Voddie Baucham, "Irreconcilable Views of Reconciliation," Grace to You, October 18, 2019, https://www.gty.org.

That's why He can emphatically tell you now that instead of being frustrated with you or feeling exasperated toward you, He instead sympathizes with your weaknesses. He feels with you and opens wide His arms with an abundance of love and compassion for you. And He calls out to you and says, "Come boldly to my throne of grace so that you may receive mercy and find grace to help you in your time of need."

So run, dear friend. Run toward your gracious and merciful High Priest and enter boldly into His presence. Don't waste another moment living under condemnation because "there is therefore now no condemnation to those who are in Christ Jesus" (Romans 8:1). Let the one who purchased you with His priceless blood and who reconciled you to Himself empower you to be His faithful ambassador and minister of reconciliation as you proclaim the glorious gospel to others.

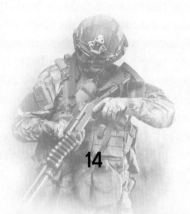

14

PUTTING A BOW
ON THE FRUIT OF THE SPIRIT

Who Controls the Controller?

I hope you're walking away from the last several chapters with a sense of clarity about what it truly means to walk in the Spirit. Clarity has a way of rousing enthusiasm in us, and this is never more fitting than when it comes to living in victory over the flesh and experiencing the euphoric freedom that comes from a harmonious existence that's in step with the Spirit of the living God. Involving ourselves in the things that God's Spirit superintends—prayer, God's Word, fellowship, and evangelism—will enable us to walk in the Spirit. Remember, the flesh will always seek to bring you under its dominion and control. It's through yielding to the Spirit's governance over your life that you will be able to live in union with Christ and resist the lusts of the flesh: "Put on the Lord Jesus Christ, and make no provision for the flesh, to fulfill its lusts" (Romans 13:14).

I thought it would be appropriate to include this brief chapter, which will contain a very important illustration, as a way of effectively encapsulating everything that I've been trying to convey about walking in the Spirit and having victory over the flesh. As we've already seen in Galatians 5, an epic battle is constantly raging between the flesh and the Spirit. This is represented by our fallen, sinful nature and the Spirit of God, who indwells us as regenerated creatures. We're told that "these are contrary to one another so that [we] do not do the things that [we] wish" (v. 17).

When the diverse aspects of a Christian's existence are carefully examined, the types of decisions they make across the various circumstances of life will indicate who or what ultimately controls them. Every believer inevitably ends up being one of two types of people. They either are controlled by the Spirit of God and bear the fruit of the Spirit or are controlled by the flesh—typically through people, thoughts, emotions, and circumstances—and bear the fruit of the flesh.

Feeling the Flow of the Flesh Frequency

A person who is controlled by the flesh is like a television set that has multiple remote controls with codes that are set to perfectly match the code in its receptor device. This means that each one of those remotes has equal capacity to control the television in multiple ways. Let's say there were twenty such remotes with twenty different people each holding one. Can you imagine the erratic activity on that television screen if each one of those people simultaneously aimed their remotes at it and began randomly pressing buttons? Power on. Power off. Power on. Brightness. Channel 7. Channel 11. Channel 9. Power off. Power on. Volume up. Volume down. Tint. Channel 4. Color. Brightness. Channel 5, 4, 2, 13, 9, 2, 4, 89, 90, 5, 92, 89, 13, 98. Mute, unmute. Power off, power on. Volume up. Contrast, aux, DVR, power off, power on, power off, power on, power off.

Someone passing by and looking in at that television would not need to be a genius to figure out that it is under the influence of multiple remote controls. That's a perfect picture of the person who is controlled by the flesh. Imagine giving every person, thought, emotion, and circumstance in the world a remote control with codes that perfectly match the code in your heart's receptor device. And anytime a button is pushed on one of those remotes, a signal emanates that solicits a response that's in keeping with the fruit of the flesh.

For example, a person hits a Speak Rudely button on their remote, and this signals you to respond with an outburst of wrath. Then, imagine one of your thoughts presses an Entitled to Indulge in Immorality button. Now you find yourself being strongly lured toward fornication. Suddenly, one of your emotions hits an Overwhelmed and Deserving of Some Relief button. You sense a powerful current dragging you toward drunkenness. Finally, a treacherous circumstance hits the Your New Coworker Just Got the Promotion You've Always Dreamed Of button, and a volcanic pressure toward hatred, jealousy, and envy rises up inside you. If you are a person who is controlled by the flesh, then you will typically respond in obedience to every one of those signals.

Smoothly in Sync with the Spirit's Signals

In contrast, a person who is controlled by the Spirit of God is like a television set that has only one remote control in the entire universe with a code that is perfectly set to match the code in its receptor device. Under that scenario, every person, thought, emotion, and circumstance can aim thousands of remotes at the television set and press buttons endlessly. However, it will remain as quiet, serene, and undisturbed as it was before anyone walked into the room. Now, those multiple signals would have definitely hit the television set's receptor device. But because the codes don't match, the television does not respond.

That's how it is with the person who is controlled by the Spirit of God. Because in any given situation, when signals in keeping with the fruit of the flesh are fired at them, God is also pressing buttons on His master remote and is sending out signals that solicit responses that are in keeping with the fruit of the Spirit. And if a person's code in their heart's receptor device matches perfectly with the code in God's master remote, then they will respond in obedience to those signals. So in place of giving in to the pull toward fornication, they yield to God's call to faithfulness. Instead of caving to the lure of drunkenness, they surrender to the Lord's draw toward self-control. And despite the strong, magnetic force sucking them in the direction of hatred, jealousy, and envy, they gladly obey the Spirit's wooing toward love, joy, and peace.

Who Pushes Your Buttons?

Interestingly, what we as people eagerly want to be true in our lives often ends up being the furthest thing from what is true about us. Many of us love to declare that we are free people who have control over the decisions that we make. However, under closer examination, we discover that we constantly allow ourselves to be controlled by people, thoughts, emotions, and circumstances. And the proof is in the pudding. Our words often reveal the condition of our hearts. So when we say things like, "He pushes my buttons," or "She pushes my buttons," or "They push my buttons," or "That pushes my buttons," then we are revealing that we are anything but free people who have control over the decisions that we make.

Toggle Switch

Now it's very important to note that we can rapidly alternate between who controls us. On any given day, we can switch back and forth multiple times between being controlled by the flesh and by God's Spirit. This all comes down to how we choose to set the code in our heart's receptor device. How then does this all work?

It's really a matter of whether we choose to be eternally minded or earthly minded. That's why Romans 12:2 tells us, "Do not be conformed to this world, but be transformed by the renewing of your mind." Paul also drove this point home in the book of Colossians: "If then you were raised with Christ, seek those things which are above, where Christ is, sitting at the right hand of God. Set your mind on things above, not on things on the earth" (3:1–2).

There's No Dumb in Freedom

When we determine to be people who don't conform to the corrupt ways of a world that hates God and that rages against Him at every turn, then things will change in our values system. We will experience the transformative power that comes from a mind that is being reshaped into the image of Christ. Likewise, as we shift the focus of our minds from the temporal things of this fading earth to the eternal realm where Christ is and where we will eventually be, we will find ourselves unmoved by the things that once consumed us and led us into bearing the fruit of the flesh.

Remember that there are those who boast about being free, yet in reality, freedom is foreign to them. But think of the sweet life of freedom that you can experience through living under the control of God's Spirit. How liberating it is when everything around you is falling apart and every person, thought, emotion, and circumstance is raging against you, yet you walk in deep peace, calm, and self-control. All the while, you're bearing the fruit of the Spirit as you respond to the Lord's signals, and most importantly, you're walking in obedience to God, which is the ultimate definition of true freedom.

My heart's greatest desire is that you see the significant correlation between this remote-control illustration and the way that its application can give you victory over sexual sin. As a man, you will be constantly bombarded by sexually charged signals coming at you from every direction and enticing you to plunge headlong into adultery, fornication, uncleanness, lewdness, and other fruits of the flesh. If your mind is conformed to this world and is set on earthly and temporal pleasures, which are both fading and destructive, then you will yield to those signals repeatedly. However, if you are transformed by the renewing of your mind and you seek those eternal things that are above, where Christ is seated, then you will yield to God's righteousness. These emanations will lovingly draw you into bearing the fruit of the Spirit, which includes patience, goodness, faithfulness, and self-control. And what true child of God wouldn't want that?

PART 3
THE WORLD

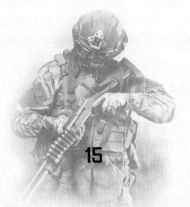

15

THE ENEMY ALL AROUND YOU

What in the World?

Satan and the flesh are our notorious enemies that are bent on destroying the slightest hint of purity in every Christian man. We've examined their insidious tactics and explored the biblical strategies through which we can have victory over their pernicious wiles. But this book would be sorely incomplete if we failed to address one more dangerous foe whose harmful effects we often overlook and minimize. We now turn our attention toward what Scripture often refers to as the world.

It must sound extremely strange to unbelievers when Christians use the word *world* in their interactions with them and say things like, "We shouldn't be of the world," or "Those are the ways of the world," or "You need to come out of the world." I would imagine that it probably comes across just as bizarre as when Christians use the word *flesh* as I mentioned in a previous chapter. Perhaps it is safe to say that both the word *world* and the biblical concept that it represents may be confusing even to some Christians.

While the Bible most certainly uses *world* when referring to the traditional understanding of the word, Scripture also uses it to depict the fallen and corrupt system of man that is in rebellion against God,

His reign as the sovereign ruler of the universe, and His transcendent, immutable moral law. This is the sort of world order that has at its helm the type of people whom the book of Romans most accurately describes:

> The wrath of God is revealed from heaven against all ungodliness and unrighteousness of men, who suppress the truth in unrighteousness, because what may be known of God is manifest in them, for God has shown it to them. For since the creation of the world His invisible attributes are clearly seen, being understood by the things that are made, even His eternal power and Godhead, so that they are without excuse, because, although they knew God, they did not glorify Him as God, nor were thankful, but became futile in their thoughts, and their foolish hearts were darkened. Professing to be wise, they became fools, and changed the glory of the incorruptible God into an image made like corruptible man—and birds and four-footed animals and creeping things.
>
> Therefore God also gave them up to uncleanness, in the lusts of their hearts, to dishonor their bodies among themselves, who exchanged the truth of God for the lie, and worshiped and served the creature rather than the Creator, who is blessed forever. Amen.
>
> For this reason God gave them up to vile passions. For even their women exchanged the natural use for what is against nature. Likewise also the men, leaving the natural use of the woman, burned in their lust for one another, men with men committing what is shameful, and receiving in themselves the penalty of their error which was due.
>
> And even as they did not like to retain God in their knowledge, God gave them over to a debased mind, to do those things which are not fitting; being filled with all unrighteousness, sexual immorality, wickedness, covetousness, maliciousness; full of envy, murder, strife, deceit, evil-mindedness; they are whisperers, backbiters, haters of God, violent, proud, boasters, inventors of evil things,

disobedient to parents, undiscerning, untrustworthy,
unloving, unforgiving, unmerciful; who, knowing the
righteous judgment of God, that those who practice such
things are deserving of death, not only do the same but also
approve of those who practice them. (Romans 1:18–32)

Paul made it clear that, at its core, the world system is one that sup-
presses the truth in unrighteousness. It's not that the truth is unknown
to them, but they intentionally push it down and replace it with blatant godlessness. This godlessness is representative of their recalcitrant
unrighteousness but is not indicative of them having no knowledge of
God's reality in the sense that they don't believe in His existence. On
the contrary, Paul emphasized the fact that God has manifested knowledge of Himself to them through His creation. And although they know
God—not in a salvific sense but from the standpoint of knowing that He
is—they choose to walk in the ways of their darkened hearts while they
refuse to glorify Him as the God they understand Him to be.

The Lord, in turn, gives the godless up to their vile passions, and
He gives them over to a debased mind. Here we find the ultimate outcome of persistent and obstinate rebellion against the God whom wicked
men know to be their Creator—the one who has given them the very
breath with which they spurn and blaspheme His holy name.

And after Paul gave an extensive list of the evil attributes and
actions that mark the haters of God, he took it one step further by rendering a harrowing description of their boundless depravity. He highlighted the fact that they not only persist in doing these wicked things
while knowing the righteous judgments of God and that they will justly
incur His wrath, but they also give approval to those who follow in their
footsteps. In other words, they propel others forward with encouragement in their evil doings. It's here that the full force of the world's diabolical sway is on display as it works to lure others into its tangled and
destructive web.

With a Friend like That, Who Needs an Enemy?

Human beings seem to have a real knack for categorization. We love
to organize things in a way that makes instant identification easy. It's

convenient to be able to say someone is a liberal, conservative, jock, goth, yuppie, gamer, introvert, extrovert, gangster, biker, or freeloader and for people to be able to immediately know the main characteristics of the person we're talking about. There are some categories that are very highly esteemed and that many take great pride in being a part of. But there is one category in particular that should make every person on the planet gladly accept a lifetime of being waterboarded daily in Guantanamo Bay rather than being a member of it. I'll let our brother James unveil this category for you: "Adulterers and adulteresses! Do you not know that friendship with the world is enmity with God? Whoever therefore wants to be a friend of the world makes himself an enemy of God" (James 4:4).

We've all heard someone say, "You don't want to be that guy's enemy." This is often said for good reasons. It's usually because that person is not someone to be trifled with. They're not some sort of weak pushover who suffers fools gladly; neither are they short on muscle or willpower when it comes to exacting retribution on their foes. But how do you even begin to compare having the most powerful and fearsome person on earth as an enemy and being at enmity with the omniscient, omnipotent, omnipresent God of the universe? How inexplicably terrifying is that?

Have you ever underestimated someone? You took one look at Bob—the short and chubby guy you got stuck with on your pickup basketball team because he was the last one left and you had last pick—and you're certain that your crew is doomed. But then he outscores everyone, is an absolute boss on defense, and leads your team to a huge victory with a 360-windmill dunk. I'm sure we've all watched at least one of those YouTube videos where someone messes with the wrong person. A little pip-squeak walks into a convenience store and pulls a knife on the dude behind the cash register. Before the wannabe thief knows it, he is regaining consciousness in the back of an ambulance with handcuffs on as the paramedics try to unravel his pretzeled body.

Some people have in their minds this celestial grandpa image of God. They think of Him as a tame, harmless, and servile butler who waits on their every beck and call, eagerly ready to fulfill all their whims and wishes. Imagine the rude awakening they will experience when they stand in the presence of the one who uses the earth as His footstool

(Isaiah 66:1) and in whose sight the nations are but a drop in a bucket and specks of dust on a scale (40:15). Where will they hide when He who is a consuming fire (Hebrews 12:29) unleashes the full force of His just wrath upon them on that unspeakably terrible day of judgment?

You would think that one would earn a moniker as serious as "enemy of God" by committing objectively severe and heinous sins. Perhaps you were surprised to find James saying that membership in this extreme category comes by way of friendship. Friendship? That's one of those words that typically buoys our hearts and triggers warm fuzzies inside us, conjuring up positive and delightful thoughts. Plus, if friendship with the world is equated to enmity with God, how does this square with Jesus being called "a friend of tax collectors and sinners" (Matthew 11:19)?

Friendship with the world does not necessarily mean having friends who are unbelievers or being friendly toward non-Christians or even living, working, and functioning amid the entrenched culture of a godless age. At its core, friendship with the world involves the adoption of and participation in the godless philosophies, ways, and activities of a corrupt system of man that is in rebellion against God.

Looking for Love in All the Wrong Places

Friendship with the world also manifests itself in a love for the world. This is something that Scripture clearly condemns: "Do not love the world or the things in the world. If anyone loves the world, the love of the Father is not in him" (1 John 2:15).

There is a massive contrast between the person who loves God and the one who loves the world. The individual who loves the Lord their God with all their heart, soul, strength, and mind will love the things He loves and approves of and will walk in glad obedience to Him in relation to those things. But the lover of the world demonstrates an affinity for the things that God hates and has forbidden in His Word. While they may claim Christ as their Savior and even refer to themselves as Christians, they have no problem thinking and behaving like the world. In fact, there's no real, distinguishable difference between them and the world, and that's because they are, in reality, of the world. They are one with that depraved, fallen, and corrupt system of man that has obstinately stiffened its neck in rebellion against almighty God, His divine reign, and His holy law. They have thrown their lot in with those who not only immerse themselves in grotesque and unbridled iniquity but also cheer on others who emulate their demonically corrupt ways.

Harmful Fun

In every man's quest for sexual purity, it's indispensable to maintain a keen awareness of this beguiling world's capacity to enchant us and lead us to the brink of the spiral of downward degradation. While seduction in both mindset and manner is a common lure, it's not typically a blatant one. More often, the world's seduction is dressed up as brilliantly liberating and enlightened philosophies and as opportunities to engage in harmless and well-deserved fun—the kind that the overwhelming majority of "respectable" people enjoy. Before we know it, as we begin to dance to this world's hypnotic drumbeat, we suddenly find ourselves entangled in the web of its traitorous friendship.

Two of the main pitfalls that we must beware of are the world's wisdom and the world's ways. We will dive deep into an exploration of these traps in the next two chapters and formulate a decimating offensive attack against them.

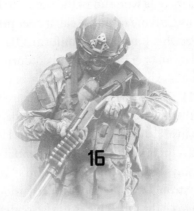

16

THE WORLD'S WISDOM

Yo! Why You Talkin' All Funny Now?

Have you ever used a cookie cutter on a delectable sheet of cookie dough? (I'm sure your mouth began watering as you read that.) How often have you dented the metal on the cookie cutter because of the hardness of the dough? Right—never. The strength of the metal against the softness of the cookie dough will always produce the same result—every single time. This world is strongly influential, and people are extremely impressionable. I'm sure you know someone who moved to another state and then magically had a different accent when you saw them again a few years later. What happened? The strong and continuous influence of the people they were surrounded by made an impression on their speech without their even realizing it.

While a change in someone's accent is inconsequential, a change in someone's perspective, outlook, and philosophy on life can be unspeakably detrimental. As the old saying goes, "Ideas have consequences." There are reasons why people in the same family typically affiliate with the same political party and why entire cities, counties, and states are designated as liberal or conservative. Proximity is a breeding ground for emulation.

Simply stated, people who run in the same circles naturally rub off on one another. In its extreme form, we call it peer pressure, and it manifests itself in the overwhelming pull to conform. Of course, there's a positive brand of emulation, peer pressure, and conformity. It's the sort that falls in line with Paul's exhortation to imitate him as he imitated Christ (1 Corinthians 11:1). And while this doesn't square with the peer pressure category—as the Lord is infinitely far from being our peer—we're exhorted in Ephesians 5:1 to be imitators of God. However, we need to identify and proactively combat any other influential element that would lead us to think in ways that are contrary to God's Word.

Paul gave a strong warning in this regard to the believers in Colossae when he wrote the following exhortation in his epistle to them: "Beware lest anyone cheat you through philosophy and empty deceit, according to the tradition of men, according to the basic principles of the world, and not according to Christ" (Colossians 2:8).

Warnings are typically given when real dangers exist. You would never tell someone not to jump too high because they may accidentally land on the moon. However, telling someone not to drive recklessly because they may get into a tragic car accident is a logical warning because there is a high probability that an accident could happen under those circumstances. Paul's urgent words aren't some token gesture coming from a sheltered man who was out of touch with reality. They are the cry of a spiritual father who had witnessed the folly of philosophy and empty deceit cheat many of his spiritual children.

Barnes' Notes on the New Testament defines the word *cheat*—or *spoil* (as the KJV translates it)—as "plunder" or "rob."[1] This is the tragic outcome for those who allow themselves to fall victim to worldly wisdom and deception.

When Simplicity Is Sweeter Than Sophistication

To fully realize the dangers associated with worldly wisdom, it's vital that we gain insight into its true essence. While we can pinpoint an array of its manifestations (and we will), understanding the root of worldly wisdom not only will help us instantly recognize when it rears its ugly head but

---

1 Albert Barnes, *Barnes' Notes on the New Testament* (Grand Rapids, MI: Kregel Publications, 1962), 1068.

will also strengthen our resistance against it when worldly wisdom seeks to invade our hearts, minds, and lives with its malice. Paul summed up the true heartbeat of worldly wisdom at the end of his exhortation in Colossians 2:8. He said that the world's wisdom is "not according to Christ." Does that sound way too simple to you? Yeah, God knew that's what we would think about it. That's why He included the following verse in His Word: "I fear, lest somehow, as the serpent deceived Eve by his craftiness, so your minds may be corrupted from the simplicity that is in Christ" (2 Corinthians 11:3).

It's important to note that even though we're now focusing on the world as a prime enemy in the life of a Christian who's in pursuit of purity, there's no question that Satan has cultivated the godless atmosphere in which the world's deceptions are rooted. Paul clearly demonstrated this in his epistle to the Ephesians as he highlighted the partnership between the world and Satan and their influence over those who are spiritually dead: "You He made alive, who were dead in trespasses and sins, in which you once walked according to the course of this world, according to the prince of the power of the air, the spirit who now works in the sons of disobedience" (Ephesians 2:1–2).

As Satan pulls the world's strings, one of his main ambitions is to corrupt our minds by drawing us away from the simplicity that is in Christ. This means that he seeks to complicate things in our hearts and lives to such a degree that he draws our attention away from Christ Himself—sometimes without us even realizing that this has happened. This all makes sense when we read 2 Corinthians 11:3 with this outlook in mind. We see, therefore, that the world's burning ambition is to cheat us through philosophies, empty deceits, traditions, and principles that are not according to Christ. In other words, all these things are contrary to the nature, teachings, commandments, and ways of Christ.

That Bully's Got a Big Ole Pulpit

The world system has a massive bully pulpit, and it has become extraordinarily adept at using it to preach its errors with extreme precision and devastating effectiveness. And it has multiple outlets through which to dispense them to its faithful disciples.

How many people do you personally know who don't own at least one, if not all, of the following devices: a television, a radio, an MP3 player, a computer, a tablet, a gaming system, or a smartphone? Yeah, me neither. These objects are mediums through which the world reaches the hearts and minds of individuals in every corner of the planet. The mediums themselves are completely neutral. There's nothing intrinsically evil about them. However, the content delivered through those mediums is a whole other matter.

So it's through movies, videos, television productions, radio talk shows, podcasts, songs, news programs, social media posts, video games, advertisements, and so on that the world disseminates its philosophies, empty deceits, traditions, and principles. And while it does it through various modern devices, let's not forget the older and more traditional mediums that are still in existence—books, magazines, newspapers, theater productions, concerts, billboards, public education, social events, and personal interaction.

Petting Bunnies Is Cool, Petting Bunnies Is Cool, Petting Bunnies Is Cool

What then are the manifestations of this worldly wisdom that is not according to Christ? You certainly don't have to look far to find them. We can find them by exploring three of the world's most popular mantras. A mantra is a phrase or slogan that one repeats as a formula or incantation, such as "I think I can; I think I can" or "Believe in yourself." These bite-size, catchy, and often-memorable mantras can be powerful and successful tools for indoctrinating others. It's the consistent and persistent repetition or demonstration of the world's statements and slogans that eventually gives them validity in people's hearts and minds. Because they become so ingrained in society's collective consciousness, to go against them almost feels like a violation of some indisputable and transcendent law.

As our examination of these three prominent worldly mantras begins, we will evaluate the essence of the message that each of them seeks to communicate and then pinpoint where they stand in direct opposition to God's Word. This will teach us how to guard ourselves against their destructive influences and remain grounded in Christ. However, don't lose sight of the fact that the actual words don't always have to be spoken in order to convey a mantra's philosophy. In other words, if "Petting bunnies is cool" were a mantra, then the constant petting of bunnies or the constant mention of petting bunnies in a positive light through various mediums would be equally as effective as verbally repeating the mantra.

"Follow Your Heart"

Let's begin with what is perhaps the most uttered mantra of the last couple of centuries: "Follow your heart."

Now doesn't that sound appealing? I'm sure you would be hard-pressed to remember a commencement speech that didn't incorporate that mantra in one form or another. It's the sort of thing that a loving grandmother or grandfather would say to one of their grandchildren as they head off to college. And it's the go-to line whenever you can't think of anything to write in your niece's or nephew's high school graduation card. But let's pause for a moment and dissect that a bit. What does "Follow your heart" even mean?

I think we gain some insight into the intended meaning of this sentiment when we recollect that it is typically followed with this statement: "It will never steer you wrong." In other words, your heart is an infallible guide that will always point you in the right direction.

Now I want you to consider the ramifications of this view. If we should always follow our heart and our heart never steers us wrong, then any kind of desire that arises within us is always a right desire that we should unquestionably fulfill. If "Follow your heart" were a valid philosophy, then every liar, thief, kidnapper, arsonist, and murderer would instantly have a legitimate excuse for their actions. "I followed my heart, your Honor, and my heart never steers me wrong."

Is this worldly philosophy according to Christ? Does it match what His Word says about the human heart? And what is Scripture referring to anyway when it talks about the heart?

When we read the word *heart* in the Bible, even though we know better, some of us subconsciously envision that organ in our chest that beats an estimated one hundred thousand times per day and pumps more than seventy-five gallons of blood through our body every hour. While that organ is extremely important to sustaining our life, biblically speaking, the heart, which is mentioned more than a thousand times in Scripture, is the seat of the emotions, the will, the desires, and the intellect. It encompasses the whole of our inner man and represents the entirety of who we really are as spiritual beings.

While Adam and Eve were created with hearts that were perfect and untainted by sin, their act of disobedience to God's command in the garden of Eden, which led to their moral fall, dramatically altered the nature of their hearts—and the hearts of their entire progeny. Jeremiah the prophet pulled back the curtain and shined a bright light on the post-fall condition of the human heart: "The heart is deceitful above all things, and desperately wicked; who can know it?" (Jeremiah 17:9).

The heart's deceitfulness is manifested by its insidious pride. This pride "keeps *true* self-knowledge hidden—the knowledge that it is deceitful, that it is wrong when it wants to appear right. Because it actually believes itself to be truly good, the self-deceived heart tends to be cavalier and crafty about the unsavory aspects of its plans, purposes, intentions, and motivations by highlighting the more respectable and honorable ones."[2]

Jesus took things a step further and highlighted the specific sins that issue from man's corrupted heart: "From within, out of the heart of men, proceed evil thoughts, adulteries, fornications, murders, thefts, covetousness, wickedness, deceit, lewdness, an evil eye, blasphemy, pride, foolishness. All these evil things come from within and defile a man" (Mark 7:21–23).

If you knew someone who was reputed to be deceitful, wicked, prideful, foolish, and capable of murder, would you follow that person's advice and trust them to faithfully guide you through life? In contrast to the world's mantra that tells you to follow your heart because it will never steer you wrong, God's Word makes it clear that you should avoid following your heart because it will never steer you right. This is why Scripture exhorts us to both watch over our hearts and infuse them with the truth of God's Word. "Watch over your heart with all diligence, for from it flow the springs of life" (Proverbs 4:23 NASB). And elsewhere, Scripture says, "Your word I have hidden in my heart, that I might not sin against You" (Psalm 119:11).

---

2   John D. Street, *Passions of the Heart: Biblical Counsel for Stubborn Sexual Sins* (Phillipsburg, NJ: P&R Publishing, 2019), 5.

Let's never forget the commentary on the manifestation of the unbridled wickedness of man's fallen heart in the days of Noah: "The LORD saw that the wickedness of man was great in the earth, and that every intent of the thoughts of his heart was only evil continually" (Genesis 6:5).

While our hearts work in conjunction with our flesh as spiritually broken sin factories and warehouses where sin is produced and stored, we have also been given a new nature through regeneration. Therefore, that spiritual battle between the fallen nature and the new nature continually rages within us.

This is why it's crucial that we remain vigilant and sober—always evaluating our inclinations and desires in light of God's divine revelation. The crucial question that we need to ask ourselves whenever we believe we are being internally led in a certain direction is this: *Does this direction agree with the Bible, or does it go against it?*

It's extremely common for people to say that their heart told them to divorce their husband or wife (who did not violate their marital covenant), or that their heart told them that they don't need to be a part of a local church fellowship because they can just have their own personal walk with the Lord, or that their heart told them to marry an unbeliever. In reality, the only thing that truly matters is what God has already said in His inerrant and infallible Word. As God's Spirit applies His written revelation to our regenerated spirit, we can be assured that He will never contradict Himself. If someone tells you that God told them to do something that conflicts with Scripture, you can boldly tell them that God most certainly did not tell them to do that. It was the misguided counsel of their worst enemy—their godless, broken, sinful heart.

After highlighting Jeremiah 17:9, about the heart of man being "desperately wicked," Owen Strachan and Gavin Peacock gave us this keen biblical insight: "We do not love God by nature; we do not obey God by nature; further, we do not want to love or obey God."[3] Then they proceeded to elaborate on how this reality manifests itself: "James locates our 'own evil desire' as the root of sin [James 1:14]. Led by a foul mind, our heart wants something wicked, something it should not want. We

---

3   Gavin Peacock and Owen Strachan, *What Does the Bible Teach about Lust?: A Short Book on Desire* (Fearn, Ross-shire, UK: Christian Focus Publications, 2020), 58–59.

feel this, perhaps, in a flash, in an instant. We then let ourselves linger on this wicked matter (whether an image, thought, word, or anything else). We mull it over in our minds, thus allowing sin to come to term."[4]

To help give us a better understanding of how our hearts harbor another one of our great enemies—lust—here again is a little more insight from Dr. John Street: "As a sincere Christian…you must be well aware of your enemy's identity and methods. You must be willing to invade your underground shelters—your hidden areas of the heart—in order to extricate him. Lust imbeds itself within your heart behind rationalizations as you yield to its deceitful feelings of satisfaction and gratification. Eventually, lust becomes your closest companion, until you no longer view life as normal without indulging it. However, you have no one to blame but yourself for fraternizing with the enemy."[5]

Firmly resisting the world's destructive mantra "Follow your heart" is essential for your sexual purity. While it's definitely possible for you to give in to your heart's promptings to indulge in sexual immorality and believe those promptings are righteous, you'll more likely rationalize more subtle promptings that will gradually set you up for your moral fall.

- *That woman whose husband just abandoned her really needs comforting. I should go to her house and be there for her during this difficult time. There's no need for me to tell my wife about it, and she will completely understand if she ends up finding out about my selfless act.*

- *What's my former, non-Christian girlfriend been up to? I should look her up on social media so that I can know how to pray for her.*

- *Yes, I'm feeling tired and stressed as I sit in my hotel room late at night during an out-of-town business trip, but turning on the TV will really help to calm and relax me.*

- *Sure, I've struggled with looking at porn on my phone and computer multiple times in the past, but this time I'm really serious about stopping. But I can do it on my*

4   Peacock and Strachan, *What Does the Bible Teach about Lust?*, 60–61.
5   Street, *Passions of the Heart*, 64.

> own; I don't need to ask a brother to keep me account-
> able, and I certainly don't need to install accountability
> software on my devices.

- *How can masturbation be wrong if almost every man
  on the planet does it? The Bible doesn't even mention
  the word. Of course, it's wrong to lust in my heart, but
  I can masturbate without lusting. After all, it's better to
  masturbate than to actually go out and commit sexual
  sin with someone because I'm so desperate for release.*

As a man, you very well understand that those scenarios are true to life. While you may only be able to identify with one or two of them, you undoubtedly know many men who would have certainly entertained every single one.

Whatever you do, don't follow your heart. Follow the truth of God's Word. It will never steer you wrong. And here's where it steers you regarding the matter of your heart: "He who trusts in his own heart is a fool" (Proverbs 28:26).

"God Wants You to Be Happy"

If ever there were a modern-day golden calf in the form of a mantra, this would unquestionably be it: "God wants you to be happy." The sacrifices that men make on its blazing altar every day are countless, and its worshipers are passionate zealots who will stop at nothing to faithfully bow before their beloved god. If skipping a day of pursuing their own happiness were considered a sin in this religion, many would unquestionably be sinless. There's not a corner of the earth that does not contain temples to this domineering deity, and every social and private forum hosts exuberant fellowship among its enthusiastic adherents.

When people regurgitate this piece of worldly wisdom, what they're essentially doing is redefining the character, nature, and commandments of God. In the final analysis, they are committing idolatry of the highest order by reshaping God into their own image. Their blasphemous insinuation is that their personal desires and feelings are so important that the omnipotent God of the universe is willing to bow to their whims and wishes at the expense of violating all that He is in His holy essence and all that He has spoken in His Holy Word about what is righteous and good.

But is the orchestration of our personal happiness the ultimate goal on God's divine agenda? While that's obviously a rhetorical question, there's nothing rhetorical about the question that naturally follows it: What *is* the ultimate goal on God's divine agenda? Those who have not bowed the knee to Christ do not merely dislike the true answer, but they utterly despise it. And this is because they want the outcome of God's ultimate goal to belong to them. And that outcome is glorification. God's supreme intent, in and through all that He accomplishes in the universe, is the glorification of His holy and awesome name (Isaiah 42:8; John 8:50; John 12:28; Romans 11:36; 1 Corinthians 10:31; 1 Peter 4:11).

Does this not seem utterly self-serving and narcissistic of God? Would not His prime goal of glorifying Himself be the epitome of megalomania, as some have contended? The answer to this depends on whether your perspective of the nature of God and the nature of man is correct. If you somehow forget that man exists only because God willed that he exists, then it would logically follow that you would think that God should somehow share glory with him. But man seeking to share in glory that doesn't belong to him, as a created creature, not only would be a form of cosmic theft but, if permitted, would lead to man's ultimate destruction.

God is the only infinite and eternal source of all things, the singular and supreme uncaused cause of every cause in the universe. Therefore, it is only right that all glory be reserved for Him alone. And that's why He very clearly says in His Word: "I am the LORD, that is My name; and My glory I will not give to another" (Isaiah 42:8).

Man seeking even the slightest amount of God's glory for himself could be likened to a fish seeking to successfully breathe outside of water. That unnatural pursuit will lead to inevitable demise. Likewise, by attempting to share in God's glory, man is seeking to become God, and this treasonous and atrocious idolatry will bring the damning wrath of God upon the impenitent idolater. Therefore, God seeking His own glory not only conforms to that which is solely and perfectly right but is also an extension of His merciful love toward mankind.

While man's eternal happiness will be one of the by-products of the glorification of God, his temporal happiness doesn't always coincide with that supreme mission of glory. In fact, sometimes man's happiness outright clashes with God's glory because it violates God's holy nature and dictates.

The mantra "God wants you to be happy" carries with it the implication that God's blessings and approval are upon man's every action as long as man's actions are in the pursuit of what makes him happy. By this logic, everything is permissible. And here is where we find the power of this deceptive mantra leading to the justification of unlawful acts that are rooted in sexual immorality—acts such as lust, adultery, fornication, pornography, and masturbation. All these sins and more will become the passionate pursuit of those who delude themselves into believing that they actually commit these iniquities beneath the shadow of God's consenting smile.

In the divine interest of glorifying Himself, God's priority for man is not that he would be temporally happy in all things but that he would function in maximal righteousness—because righteousness glorifies God. This will often mean that man must be willing to sacrifice both legitimate and illegitimate pursuits for the sake of fulfilling God's perfect and sovereign will.

Among other things, two of the most positive results from living in step with this reality include both protection from the ravages of sinful indulgence and something that is far better than happiness: the unspeakable joy of being a vessel of honor through which God receives glory. Against this magnificent backdrop, we can see the worldly wisdom that says "God wants you to be happy" for the foolish and shallow nonsense that it really is.

"You Only Live Once"

I can't help but wonder how many lives have been tragically shipwrecked on the shores of this misleading mantra: "You only live once," a.k.a. YOLO. What's even more terrifying is to think of the severe accounting that many souls will give on the day of judgment for having danced to the beat of this foolish philosophy's drum.

Good ole YOLO has given birth to many well-intentioned adventurers. "This is the only life I'll ever be able to live, so I should do some rock climbing, parasailing, and traveling," they say. While still misguided, this is really no biggie. But then there are those who also drink at the well of "Life is short." While this related mantra could actually be spiritually beneficial, when it joins forces with its big sister YOLO, it becomes a catalytic accelerator that puts the pursuit of outright hedonism into overdrive.

While not everyone who lives by this motto explicitly denies the existence of God or believes that there is no life after this earthly one has passed, most, nonetheless, practically live like atheists and materialists. They prove where their heart truly is by where they have stockpiled their treasure. They are bottomless-pit consumers, pleasure-seeking gallivanters, and revelers in all things frivolous.

It would seem logical that man's acknowledgment of his mortal nature would lead him to treasure his transient life, to contemplate the possibility of the eternal, and to sincerely seek after the type of spiritual truth that would help him make sense of a universe that is uniformly marked with divine fingerprints. While some certainly end up traveling this path and discovering the glorious gospel (or succumbing to a false form of spirituality), most will choose a haphazard life of reckless abandon, frantically indulging in everything possible before it's lights out.

Yes, we do only live once—on this side of eternity. But if we have undergone the new birth and have been transformed by the redeeming power of the gospel, we will live again (John 11:25). It's true that we will die in this temporal world. However, if we fail to repent and place our faith in Christ, we will die again through what the Bible refers to as "the second death" (Revelation 21:8). This type of death will be experienced in a place of eternal and conscious torment called the lake of fire, where we will forever pay for our unforgiven sin and rebellion against our holy God (vv. 7–8).

If You Eat Too Many Carrots, Your Skin Will Turn Orange

While these three mantras are but a small sampling of the type of worldly wisdom that constantly surrounds Christians, they nonetheless help to drive the broader point home. Unless God's people are determined to cultivate a biblically grounded perspective on every aspect of life and immerse themselves in the sincere and passionate pursuit of Christ and His eternal kingdom, they will inevitably find themselves susceptible to the influences of the world's foolish and destructive philosophies. While a great portion of the planet's population is ignorant of what real wisdom is—some, I'm sure, concluding that *wisdom* is just the name of a tooth—the Christian's greatest weapon against the wisdom of the world is to walk in the fear of the Lord, which is the beginning of wisdom (Proverbs 9:10).

As Christians go about life on this planet, it's inevitable that they will hear the chants of the world's wisdom and see that misguided wisdom lived out before their eyes. Paul the Apostle implied this when he said the following about interacting with the ungodly: "I wrote to you in my epistle not to keep company with sexually immoral people. Yet I certainly did not mean with the sexually immoral people of this world, or with the covetous, or extortioners, or idolaters, since then you would need to go out of the world" (1 Corinthians 5:9–10).

However, every believer must examine his own heart to see if he has allowed himself to be influenced by worldly wisdom. I explained earlier in this chapter that the world exerts its influence on people's minds by dispensing its mantras and philosophies through multiple media platforms and other types of outlets. If Christians fall into the habit of indiscriminately immersing themselves in the worldly content that flows from these sources, it's inevitable that they will allow worldly thinking to guide their lives. While in the next chapter we will further explore how this affects one's behavior, I'd like to end this discussion here with a sobering quote from R. Kent Hughes's powerful book *Disciplines of a Godly Man*: "Men, it is impossible for you to maintain a pure mind if you are a television-watching, internet-surfing, video-game-playing 'couch potato.' In one week, you will watch more murders, adulteries, and perversions than our grandfathers read about in their entire lives… No man who allows the rottenness of R-rated movies and shows, the various 'soft-core' pornography magazines, and suggestive digital images to flow through their house and mind will escape sensuality."[6]

---

6   R. Kent Hughes, *Disciplines of a Godly Man*, updated ed. (Wheaton, IL: Crossway, 2019), 41–42.

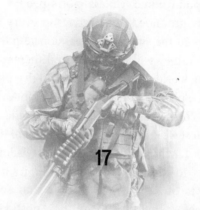

17

THE WORLD'S WAYS

Keep Your Finger off the Zoom Button

I had been going there to share the gospel almost every Friday night for a couple of years, but this particular evening felt very different. As I walked between the towering buildings along the famed Third Street Promenade in Santa Monica, I felt like I was turning into the real-life Incredible Shrinking Man. From the emotion-stirring music to the massive, deafening crowds, to the exuberant street performers, to the glamorously dressed people strutting in and out of swanky restaurants and high-end shops, to the shiny super cars that were zooming by—the world, in all its ostentatious pomp and glory, was out in full force. I was suddenly daunted by its overpowering bigness, and I felt like I was a tiny ant crawling about in the shadow of Mount Everest. I was gripped by a palpable sense of insignificance and powerlessness as I walked around trying to hand out tracts and share the gospel with others. But then I realized what my problem was. I was so focused on the world that it became enormous in my mind, and this made me lose sight of the greatness of my God.

I loved the classic black-and-white *King Kong* and *Godzilla* movies when I was a kid. I was mesmerized by how both monsters crushed houses, cars, and trees beneath their feet and how they stood almost as tall as skyscrapers. While I knew the creatures weren't real and that actors in costumes were playing them, my young mind couldn't comprehend how the filmmakers had found such giant men for those roles. But when I grew up, I was enlightened to the splendid glories of movie magic. I discovered the revolutionary realities of the zoom button.

When a camera lens zooms in closely on a movie set where the director desires to create the effect of size alteration, the zoom completely skews the viewer's perspective of reality and creates a proportion illusion. I came to understand that if the camera panned out, the gargantuan beasts on my television screen would appear as they are in truth—two average blokes in monkey and lizard suits stomping around in a sandbox filled with Tonka trucks, Hot Wheels cars, dollhouses, and miniature-scale replicas of giant buildings.

Aided by our fallen, sinful nature, our heart's default setting is always on maximum zoom in the direction of our native home. Our natural inclination is to fixate on a world that stands ready and willing to scratch us where we itch—dishing up the dainty delicacies that satisfy our sinful cravings. When our focus is properly adjusted on our infinite God and His eternal purposes and we look down on this world and all that it contains from His lofty, divine heights, we see not only this planet but also the entire universe and everything in it as the finite and fading specks that they actually are. We then remember that this same God is our Lord and Redeemer and the one who actually indwells us, making us temples of His Spirit. This infuses us with a blazing passion to prize, prioritize, and pursue Him and His interests above all else.

However, the more we fixate on this world, the larger and more significant it becomes in our eyes and the more minimized our God, His kingdom, and the things of eternity become to us. This then triggers a drift from worship, an abandonment of God's presence, a diminished passion for holiness, and a life devoid of discipline and self-control. Before we know it, we are no longer walking in the pure and undefiled faith highlighted in James 1:27. In contrast to James' exhortation, we tragically find ourselves stained and spotted by the world.

Walk This Way, Talk This Way

When a Christian's perception of reality becomes skewed, the repercussions can be both crippling and devastating. Being surrounded by a world and a world system that loom large—even in the imagination—can create a sense of resignation that we can't possibly resist the sinful temptations that the world offers. This can lead to the defeatist mindset that says, "If you can't beat them, join them." At this unfortunate juncture, walking in the world's wisdom inevitably turns into living according to the world's ways.

The world's culture is alive and well, thriving, expanding, and successfully serving its own purposes as it proliferates across the planet and leaves a trail of destruction in its wake. Yes, it's certainly alive and well as it causes death and sickness in everyone it touches—much like a virus—often moving invisibly and undetected from one host to another.

As we now examine some of the specific ways of the world, I pray that we're willing to genuinely humble our hearts and ask ourselves the hard questions about the areas in our lives that may have been tainted by the ways of the world. As we did in our examination of the world's wisdom, we will examine three of the world's most prominent ways.

Fitting In: Leave That Round Hole Alone, Mr. Square Peg

No one wants to look like a weirdo or be the odd one out. While Hollywood celebrities are undoubtedly trendsetters in many respects, keep in mind that they, too, are trying to fit in. They buy the popular name-brand cars and wear the most fashionable outfits. They also get hair transplants, plastic surgery, and liposuction for a reason. Fitting in is a big part of the world's culture. This is tied into a desire for acceptance and validation. In most cases, mimicking external elements of this sort isn't a big deal, but there's a massive problem when striving for acceptance crosses over into compromising righteousness in order to score an attaboy from a world that fundamentally opposes everything that God stands for.

Imagine these scenarios: Most of your coworkers are going to a wild concert, and they invite you to join them, assuring you that there will be plenty of single women at the event looking to connect with an eligible bachelor like yourself. You had already turned them down for two other concerts and a weekend of club-hopping and gambling in Las Vegas. At this point, you sense if you say no to this, you're definitely going to become an outcast in the company.

An old friend from high school is getting married, and he asks you to be one of the groomsmen at his wedding. You're honored and gladly accept. The bachelor party is scheduled for the next weekend, and the boys have secured a couple of exotic dancers. They are also planning to booze it up and watch some raunchy movies. Skipping out on the party could cost you the friendship.

You've been single for a very long time and have been intensely struggling with loneliness. Most of your friends are either dating, engaged, or married. There are no girls at church or work who show any interest in you, and you find this to be both frustrating and deeply painful. On top of that, your unsaved parents keep hounding you to finally get married, and that's putting a lot of pressure on you. An attractive woman at the gym starts paying attention to you and is even a bit flirtatious. This feels good. The only problem is that she's not a Christian. After about a month of regular interaction with her, she invites you to coffee. You begin to question if it really is unbiblical to be in a relationship with an unbeliever. You fear that if you don't accept her invitation, you might blow your chance of finding a soulmate, disappoint your parents, and continue living in loneliness.

You made a few new friends through the local softball league that you recently joined, and after a couple months of getting to know each other, they invite you and your girlfriend to join them on an annual camping trip they go on with their girlfriends. You don't own a tent, and neither does your girlfriend. One of your new buddies tells you not to worry about it because he has a few extra tents and would have you both covered. When you arrive at the campground, you find that your friend arrived before the rest of the group and has even set up the tents he brought—one for him and his girlfriend and one for you and yours. You swallow hard. You force a smile and attempt to conceal your shock. After a few minutes of trying to calm your internal panic, you discreetly take him aside and ask him if some of the others might be bringing an extra tent with them. He looks a bit puzzled and tells you that it wouldn't make any sense for them to do that since they already have one tent per couple. It somehow slipped your mind that this is how the world rolls. When you discuss it with your girlfriend, she tells you it's no big deal, that she's fine with the arrangement, and that you'll both make sure to maintain self-control. Do you go along with it, or do you object and rock the boat—risking looking like some crazy religious fanatic in front of your newfound friends?

While these particular examples related to sexual temptations are fictitious, we know that Christian men face similar scenarios in the real world every single day. Whether it's attending a godless concert where ungodly people abound, going to a lust-filled bachelor party, dating someone who doesn't love Christ, or being in a compromising position with a girlfriend, our options are still the same: either we will follow the ways of the world, which tell us to conform at any cost in order to be accepted, or we will instead seek to honor the Lord and do what's right in His sight.

Christians are sometimes shocked that the people of this world reject them and are even hateful toward them. But this shouldn't surprise believers at all. If we are truly disciples of Christ, then why would we expect people to treat us any differently than they treated our Savior? Jesus already told us that this is exactly how things would be: "If the world hates you, you know that it hated Me before it hated you. If you were of the world, the world would love its own. Yet because you are not of the world, but I chose you out of the world, therefore the world hates you" (John 15:18–19).

So Jesus made it abundantly clear that being hated or rejected by the world because of our pursuit of Christ is par for the course. What our Lord said makes perfect sense. If the God-hating, righteousness-rejecting, sin-loving world vigorously opposed Him, why would its citizens treat His followers any differently? Those who do have the world's full acceptance might need to check themselves and examine if they are truly walking in total surrender to Christ in every aspect of their lives.

Let's consider for a moment what the early disciples endured for Jesus' sake. And as we do this, it's important to bear in mind that they did these things while living in a culture that placed a high premium on conformity. Community and being an accepted part of that community were everything in that era. It was certainly not the age of rugged individualism, when being a maverick was all the rage. What one was willing to endure for the sake of another directly correlated to the level of one's commitment to that person. Let's begin by looking at Paul's description of what he and the apostles endured for the sake of Christ:

> I think that God has displayed us, the apostles, last, as men condemned to death; for we have been made a spectacle to the world, both to angels and to men. We are fools for Christ's sake, but you are wise in Christ! We are weak, but you are strong! You are distinguished, but we are dishonored! To the present hour we both hunger and thirst, and we are poorly clothed, and beaten, and homeless. And we labor, working with our own hands. Being reviled, we bless; being persecuted, we endure; being defamed, we entreat. We have been made as the filth of the world, the offscouring of all things until now. (1 Corinthians 4:9–13)

That hardly sounds like people who were striving to fit in and angling for acceptance. Think of some of the verbiage that Paul used to paint a picture of how he and the apostles were viewed and treated: "a spectacle to the world," "fools," "dishonored," "reviled," "persecuted," "defamed," "the filth of the world." That is a clear indication that they were truly living for an audience of One and they were willing to risk both their reputation and the enjoyment of passing worldly pleasures in order to honor and glorify God through surrender and obedience.

The response of the apostles after the powerful religious leaders of their day commanded them to stop preaching about Christ has often humbled and convicted me: "Peter and the other apostles answered and said: 'We ought to obey God rather than men'" (Acts 5:29). We would do well to learn from their example. While others may not be commanding us to stop preaching about Jesus, the pressure that their approval or disapproval exudes can surely tempt us to compromise our obedience to Christ when it comes to sexual purity. We must be resolved to say that we will continue obeying God's Word rather than caving to the influences of man.

But what's even more amazing than their response to the command of their captors was the attitude of the apostles after those same men beat them for their commitment to Jesus: "They departed from the presence of the council, rejoicing that they were counted worthy to suffer shame for His name. And daily in the temple, and in every house, they did not cease teaching and preaching Jesus as the Christ" (Acts 5:41–42).

Wow! Fathom that. After being imprisoned, beaten, and threatened, the apostles went on their way rejoicing. Rejoicing? Really? Someone unfriends or unfollows us on social media because of a Bible verse we posted, and we curl up into a ball and cry out, "The sky is falling!" The apostles actually considered themselves honored that God allowed them to suffer shame for His name. It's interesting that the word *worthy* is used to describe their perception of the shame that the Lord graced them with. This means that they would have viewed themselves as unworthy if they had not been permitted to endure the world's scorn for the name of Christ.

While the world heaps its shame on us, we have nothing to be ashamed of because we are walking in righteousness. It was a wise man who said that "Christians have nothing to be ashamed of apart from sin." Peter gave us clear marching orders when it comes to the type of attitude that we're to have in the face of the world's afflictions: "Let none of you suffer as a murderer, a thief, an evildoer, or as a busybody in other people's matters. Yet if anyone suffers as a Christian, let him not be ashamed, but let him glorify God in this matter" (1 Peter 4:15–16).

There's only one thing worse than being ashamed of suffering as a Christian—being ashamed of the Christ of Christianity. The words that our Savior spoke about this should make every Christian shudder: "Whoever is ashamed of Me and My words in this adulterous and sinful generation, of him the Son of Man also will be ashamed when He comes in the glory of His Father with the holy angels" (Mark 8:38).

The atrociousness of being ashamed of Christ is amplified all the more when we consider the audience before whom we are displaying this shame. It makes perfect sense that, in the presence of impeccable holiness, the spotless Lamb of God would be ashamed of those who were ashamed of Him before a wicked world.

In contrast to a life that strives to fit in with the world, let's pursue a different type of "fitting" that God's Word commends. It's the kind of "fitting" that is suitable for those of us who have been called as saints—as ones who are set apart and whose lives are to be so diametrically opposed to the ways of the world that not even the slightest hint of sexual sin is so much as whispered among us: "Fornication and all uncleanness or covetousness, let it not even be named among you, as is fitting for saints" (Ephesians 5:3).

Let's make pleasing the Lord our greatest ambition because that's the true hallmark of a child of God: "Do I now persuade men, or God? Or do I seek to please men? For if I still pleased men, I would not be a bondservant of Christ" (Galatians 1:10).

The Pursuit of Pleasure: If It Feels Good, Think Twice Before You Do It

The human body is truly a masterpiece of ingenuity and design. We've touched on that already in this book, and we'll explore it further in upcoming pages. However, there is one aspect of our makeup as marvelously fashioned creatures that I can't help but highlight here. It's one that adds zest and flavor to life. It's an element that transforms a tiny 1950s black-and-white television set into an IMAX 3D theater. It turns bland egg whites into Belgian Godiva truffles, and it magically morphs a free set of airline headphones into Dolby surround sound speakers—with subwoofers. In case you haven't figured it out yet, I'm talking about pleasure. Imagine how dull and predictable life would be without it.

When we think of pleasure in the context of sex, thoughts of excessive debauchery and wanton immorality often come to mind. Obviously, our aim is to avoid diving into these sorts of sinful excesses. However, we must realize that the world has normalized other unwise and possibly harmful entanglements as a part of its culture and that, sadly, many Christians have adopted them. While these things can definitely become sinful in and of themselves (depending on some specific factors), they can, at the very least, become the gateway to sexual sin and lead us into it in progressive stages.

In concert with our imagination and our emotions, pleasure is completely sensory. It's through the portals of taste, touch, smell, sight, and sound that we experience pleasure. The way of the world is to interact with these portals as pleasure suppliers in ways and degrees that are dictated by the world's relativistic standards. This is especially true when it comes to touch, sight, and sound. In other words, feel, look at, and listen to whatever you would like and however much of it you would like as long as you think it's right for you. This is where the individual, independent of the standards of morality that God has established, becomes the sole arbiter of what is right and wrong for him. (Recall what we have already explored in part one regarding deification.)

Here's how this all plays out when it comes to the first worldly entanglement we'll be examining. It's hard to imagine that there was a time when there were no such things as theaters and televisions. And after those technologies came into existence, who could ever have fathomed the emergence of computers and smartphones? It's now even become hard for us to remember a time when on-demand videos, streaming services, and online video platforms (like YouTube) didn't exist.

The pleasure that the mind and body derive from sight is far greater than most people realize. It's true, as Ecclesiastes 1:8 says, that "the eye is not satisfied with seeing." This means there is no limit to man's insatiable appetite to look at desirable objects. And the revenue-driven world is all too keen to supply the brightest and shiniest eye-catching things to satisfy every person's distinct viewing preferences. Pardon my use of hyperbole, but with video screens now plastered over almost every square inch of the planet, you can't really escape them. But the screens—whether in public, in our homes, in our offices, or in our hands—aren't the problem. The problem is what those screens often display and how Christians are buying into the way of the world, which says that it's fine to watch whatever you want to your heart's content.

When a Christian man spends vast amounts of time in front of a television set or a giant screen in a movie theater; when he takes in hours of video content through his smartphone, tablet, and computer; and when the images and sounds that he's absorbing through those mediums are filled with profanity, vileness, blasphemy, lust, pride, greed, and gratuitous violence, it's impossible for him to walk away unscathed. Now add countless images of deliberately provocative and scantily dressed women, a plethora of illicit innuendoes, and a barrage of steamy sex scenes, and how strong do you think he will stand when faced with the sexual temptations that will bombard him on a daily basis?

Not only are we told in Scripture that "the eye is not satisfied with seeing," but the rest of Ecclesiastes 1:8 says, "Nor the ear filled with hearing." It's rare anymore to see people in public without sporting earbuds or headphones. Whether walking down the street, exercising at the gym, waiting to be seen in a doctor's office, lounging around at the park, or shopping at the mall or supermarket, audio content is constantly flowing into people's heads. And similar to the impact that comes from what people intake through their eyes, what we listen to can greatly impact how we behave.

If you want to know how much music influences the emotions, just watch what happens when a crowd is dancing at a party and the tunes suddenly cut out. Everyone immediately stops midmotion, and the embarrassed grins that involuntarily appear on their faces betray how silly they feel on the inside. It's difficult to explain the mechanics behind it, but God has hardwired us to be musical beings, and sometimes we can't help but react to the rhythmic melodies that penetrate our souls.

I remember once watching a video that showed a scary scene from a classic movie. However, the fear-inducing music in the original version was replaced with cheerful, upbeat music. And then a fun-filled and joyous scene from another movie appeared, but the bouncy music was replaced with sinister horror music. I couldn't believe how much the audio switch altered my feelings and perceptions when I watched each scene.

Music is indeed powerful, and that can be a very positive thing. However, there's something else that could have an even greater influence over us for good or bad. I'm referring to the lyrics that often accompany music. Songs are packed with messages that reflect deeply held worldviews and philosophies. They can shape our thinking and evoke a whole host of different reactions in us. I can't help but wonder what a person from the 1940s would feel if they traveled in time and compared the lyrics found in some of our contemporary songs with the ones from their era. Utter shock would probably be putting it mildly.

It's appalling to consider how so much worse song lyrics have gotten since the first Parental Advisory labels were slapped on CD and cassette covers in the 1990s. As profane as things were then, most of the "bad" songs from that time sound like innocent lullabies when contrasted with what's being released today. And yet there are many who contend that they only listen to songs for the music and aren't really influenced by the lyrics. Not only does that fly in the face of common sense and scientific facts, but listening to filthy lyrics violates explicit commands of Scripture, which we will shortly explore in this chapter. Think of the countless violent crimes, murders, and suicides that have been directly linked to specific songs. Unlike a movie that someone may watch anywhere from one time to a handful of times, it's not unusual for someone to listen to certain songs hundreds and maybe even thousands of times over the course of their lifetime. How is it possible to hear words repeated that many times and not in some way be influenced by them— or at the very least become desensitized to the egregious messages that some of those words convey?

The audio realm obviously extends far beyond the world of music. Radio outlets and podcast platforms supply an endless array of auditory offerings to satisfy avid listeners of every stripe. From talk show hosts to comedians, to political commentators, to celebrated influencers, everyone has something to say—and a lot of it. It brings to mind Proverbs 10:19, which tells us that "in the multitude of words, sin is not lacking." Once again, think about the lewd, crass, unclean, and unwholesome content that's often associated with programs of this sort.

Sometimes we end up listening to the voices of the people on the other side of our speakers more than we do those of our wife, children, friends, and spiritual mentors. And most of the things those voices are telling us do nothing to nurture our souls or benefit our minds. When it comes down to it, much of it is just empty noise that ends up darkening our hearts and marring our consciences. Now that's tragic.

There's one more pleasure that I'm compelled to mention at this juncture, and I do so not out of a personal desire but from sheer necessity. This pet pleasure has reached epic heights of popularity—especially in the last decade. If you haven't guessed by now, I'm talking about gaming.

When I was a teenager in the late '80s and early '90s, the NES (Nintendo Entertainment System) was the hottest thing on the market. It made my elementary school days of playing *Space Invaders* on my Atari 2600 feel like something from ancient times. But now, the PlayStation and Xbox systems, with their mind-blowing graphics, hyperrealism, and virtual reality integration, have gone far beyond anything I could have dreamed or imagined. But by the same token, so has the content. This has truly become an arena where the demonically perverse and twisted elements of man's fallen, sinful nature are explicitly manifested. Unbridled foulness is running amok in the expansive world of video gaming by glorifying criminal activities and allowing the player to revel in the most senseless and brutal violence, drug use, and perverse sexual encounters.

Although our focus has been on indecent video game content, we must never forget another troubling aspect associated with that whole realm: the inordinate amount of time that people devote to what, for many, has become an intensely addictive pastime. It's not uncommon for young men to spend thirty to forty hours per week sitting in a trancelike state, staring at a screen while their fingers incessantly move on the controller to manipulate the action on the screen.

What's even more disturbing is that this is not confined to teenage boys, but it's also true of grown men in their twenties, thirties, forties, and beyond. Multitudes of men with careers and a wife and children are committing almost as much time to playing games as they are to their careers—and certainly much more than they're devoting to their families. With this massive volume of time committed to such a frivolous pursuit, there isn't much energy or focus left over for the cultivation of the soul. Many men underestimate the harmful effects that such an activity can have on their spiritual life. And whenever someone challenges them about their lack of discipline in connection with their faith, they unbelievably say that they just don't have the time.

While we can ask a thousand questions and make ten thousand comments about what's appropriate to watch, listen to, and play, what really matters is what God's Word has to say about the illicit pleasures that entice Christians to dive headlong into following the way of the world in this arena. And for this we turn our attention toward Philippians 4:8: "Brethren, whatever things are true, whatever things are noble, whatever things are just, whatever things are pure, whatever things are lovely, whatever things are of good report, if there is any virtue and if there is anything praiseworthy—meditate on these things."

This isn't about legalistic rules not to watch movies, television programs, and videos. It has nothing to do with imposing laws that forbid Christians to listen to secular music and talk radio. And it's certainly not an attempt to label gaming as an evil activity. In fact, recreation is both healthy and necessary. The mind and the body were designed to rest, to disconnect from intense concentration on work, and to recharge by allowing the senses to engage in enjoyable and leisurely activities. These activities can most certainly include the marvelous and brilliant creations of man that we've discussed. But the question is whether the content associated with these activities aligns with the things God's Word calls His people to meditate on.

This laudable meditation list prescribed by Paul reveals God's best for the hearts and minds of His people. And doesn't it make perfect sense that the designer of our hearts and minds would know better than anyone else which things are most conducive to our inner flourishing? Truth, nobility, justice, purity, loveliness, reputability, virtue, and praiseworthiness are all good for the nurturing of our souls.

There are enough distasteful things in this world that we can't avoid seeing and hearing. And there are things that we should choose to look at and listen to that don't align with what Paul outlined in Philippians 4:8. I'm referring to stories of unjust wars, abuse, oppression, injustice, tyranny, and the like. However, our intentional encounter with these sorts of things should always carry with it some kind of redemptive purpose or a motive to bring a solution to these ills by better understanding them—but never for the purpose of frivolous entertainment. Imagine the difference it would make in the world if every believer used Philippians 4:8 to evaluate everything that they had the option of looking at and listening to.

It's easy at this juncture to assume that while men may listen to and meditate on inappropriate things, it won't hurt their pursuit of purity as long as those things are not sexual in nature. But this is not necessarily true. The carelessness and lackadaisical attitude associated with unfettered viewing and listening habits—even if it is not technically of X-rated content—not only makes men more susceptible to crossing into pornographic sites, but it also lowers their ability to resist engaging in physical acts of sexual immorality.

A man who does not weigh his listening and viewing choices on the scale of God's Word may also have deeper issues to face. Such careless habits of entertainment indicate a heart that has loosened its grip on the fear of God and diverted its gaze from eternal matters. It implies an adoption of the world's ways and an idolatrous pursuit of pleasure at any cost.

"My Body, My Choice": What a Stupid Mantra

"My body, my choice." When we hear this mantra, our thoughts immediately go to the abortion issue. However, the mindset and philosophy that fuel the sentiments of "My body, my choice" spill over into many other areas of life. The way of the world is to seek complete independence from God and to claim total autonomy over one's life, which includes one's body and what one does with it. There was a time when society, at least publicly, praised the virtue of sexual purity. Premarital sex was frowned upon, and an unmarried couple living together was virtually unheard of. In the rare cases where cohabitation did happen, the couple would usually lie and say they were husband and wife to avoid a scandal. Not only have both premarital sex and living together without getting married become completely normalized in our current culture, but it's not uncommon for couples to unashamedly ask a pastor to officiate at their wedding while unflinchingly disclosing that they're living together— and by implication, fornicating. In fact, they're completely shocked and offended when anyone even hints that there's something inappropriate about that.

While every genuinely saved Christian acknowledges that fornication is a sin, the world's insistence on bodily autonomy can affect the way we think. However, we justify this attitude by contrasting our sin with that of the world. We try to appease our consciences by appealing to the minimalistic standard of not going as far as the world does. The justification goes something like this: *Almost all my unbelieving friends regularly have sex with their girlfriends. While my girlfriend and I do passionately make out and get a little touchy sometimes, at least we've never had sex.*

But isn't it tragic when God's children live by the minimalistic standard of getting as close as we can to the boundary line of sin and compromise without crossing it? Shouldn't our hearts long to get as far away from sin as possible? And instead of using the world's ways as our measuring rod, shouldn't we instead be asking ourselves what God's Word has to say on the matter? Because it's quite likely that many of the physical activities that some believers accept by minimalist standards in their premarital relationships are actually sinful in the sight of God.

Now here's the spot where some of you will be tempted to throw this book across the room, then punch it a few times before shredding it in the garbage disposal. And I'm sure thoughts of putting a picture of my face on a dartboard will definitely cross your mind. But before you do all that, I appeal to you to hear me out.

If you've read everything I've written up to this point, it's a good indication that you sincerely desire to honor the Lord by walking in sexual purity. This means we're on the same page. I wrote this book because I want to help you in this endeavor, and I'm going out on a limb by saying some very unpopular things that I believe men need to hear. I have no interest in running your life and telling you what to do. I just want to give you some important points to think about.

Remember that it's easy to interpret sexual actions based on whether the Bible explicitly says they are sin. But when we do this, we end up tossing out the use of discernment and wisdom, and in so doing, we can find ourselves engaging in things that may not be technically labeled as sin but that can definitely lead us into sin.

So here it goes. I want you to honestly ask yourself if it's wise for a recovering alcoholic to spend time in a bar and keep bottles of beer stocked in his fridge. How about a person who's seeking to repent of gluttony? Do you think it's prudent for him to go to all-you-can-eat buffets and hang out around ice-cream parlors? Should former gambling addicts frequent casinos? Should someone who's trying to quit smoking stop in at smoke shops? Should recovering spendthrifts go to the mall on Black Friday?

Now it's obvious that it's not illegal for people to visit any of those places. But wouldn't it be tragically sad for individuals who have had the problems I highlighted to use the legality of these actions as their justification for participating in them? "It's fully within my legal right to go to a bar; therefore, I'm going there." But is it healthy? Is it best? Is it wise? And wouldn't it be more likely that someone recovering from or struggling with an addiction would relapse if they insist on exercising their legal right to go to these places?

Perhaps you're thinking that I'm taking things a bit too far by drawing an analogy between addictions and one's natural desire to engage in certain intimate activities with a girlfriend or fiancée. I'll concede that no analogy is perfect, and they all end up breaking down at some point, but let's not forget all that we've already explored regarding Satan's schemes, the battle between our flesh and the Spirit, and the constant lure of the world. All this should be enough to tell you that it's not a far stretch to compare the dangers of hanging around places that can supply a fix for your addictions to the dangers of getting too affectionately close with your significant other before you're married.

And what does real-life experience show us? How many Christian couples have started with passionate kissing and close bodily contact and have not gone further? And while most would have unquestionably gone further physically, do you think that any such Christian couple who refrained from physical sin didn't at least go further in their hearts and minds?

So I would encourage you to give this some serious thought. If you truly believe what Paul said in 1 Corinthians 7:1–2, that because of sexual immorality, it's good for a man not to touch a woman (meaning in a sexually arousing way), and if you acknowledge that Jesus equated lust in a person's heart to adultery, wouldn't common sense conclude that the optimal choice is to refrain from passionate kissing and close bodily contact? Is it unbiblical? Can we find a passage that specifically says don't kiss your girlfriend before you're married and don't engage in long hugs where your bodies are pressed up against one another? Does Scripture say that you can't be in a house or room alone together for extended periods of time or that it's forbidden to sit in a parked car late at night for hours on end with the seats reclined as you lie in one another's arms? No. You won't find any Scripture passages that explicitly forbid these things. But to harken back to the questions we considered earlier in this chapter, are these situations healthy? Are they best? Are they wise? I'll let you answer those questions.

If we're honest with ourselves, it's at this juncture that we are most tempted to adopt the way of the world that says, "My body, my choice." If we don't say it with our words, our attitude is likely to convey, *God doesn't strictly forbid me in the Bible to do this, so I can do this. I want to do this, and I'm going to do this.* Setting aside any discussion about potentially sinning against one's conscience and that whatever we do not do from faith is sin, let me say that you're right. The Bible does not strictly forbid these things, and you can, in fact, do them.

My sincere prayer for you, if you choose to do these things, is that you get to the other side of your participation in these activities without having ventured into any sin. My ultimate hope for you, however, is that you won't stop at that minimalistic standard of asking if you have a right to partake in these activities. I hope you'll probe deeper into your soul and ask, *Is doing this healthy? Is it best for me and for the person I love? Is it wise? And will it most glorify God, guard me from sin, and keep me from leading into sin the person whom I claim to love?* After all, it's actually not your body: "Flee sexual immorality. Every sin that a man does is outside the body, but he who commits sexual immorality sins against his own body. Or do you not know that your body is the temple of the Holy Spirit who is in you, whom you have from God, and you are not your own? For you were bought at a price; therefore glorify God in your body and in your spirit, which are God's" (1 Corinthians 6:18–20).

Paul prefaced these words with profound truth when he said the following in verse 12: "All things are lawful for me, but not all things are profitable" (NASB1995). May we care enough to consider the significance of this sobering reality.

As I close this chapter, let me tell you that I've seen couples who chose not to save close bodily contact and their first kiss for their wedding day. And I've seen the resulting ravages of that decision time and time again—almost without exception. But there's something else I've seen *completely* without exception—the joy, sweetness, freedom, and long-lasting benefits for every couple I've known who has chosen to take the path less traveled. After all, sexual purity maintained between a man and a woman before marriage is a gift that can never be taken away from them once they've entered marriage. And it's a priceless gift that keeps on giving.

We focused on some of the key ways of the world with the aim of detecting them and understanding them. We did this for the ultimate purpose of learning how important it is to no longer zoom in on the world and, therefore, magnify it in our hearts and minds. Rather, we discovered that our ambition should be to zoom out from it and see things from the standpoint of our great and awesome God—consequently magnifying Him and His ways and, in turn, minimizing this fading world and its influence on our lives. As we resist the world's ways in the pursuit of pleasure, the ambition to fit in, and the commitment to claim autonomy over what we do with our bodies, may God strengthen us to recognize that only His ways are right and true, for as His Word powerfully declares, "There is a way which seems right to a man, but its end is the way of death" (Proverbs 14:12).

PART 4

SIX CS AND A NOPE

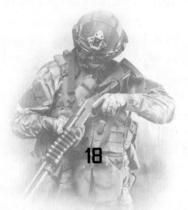

18

CREATION

WIELD WONDERS AS WELLSPRINGS FOR WORSHIP, NOT WEAPONS FOR WOUNDING

Six Cs to Succeed

So here's where things begin to get very practical. Of course, we've covered a number of practical elements associated with combating the main tactics of Satan, the flesh, and the world, but in this final section, we're going to step things up a few notches. I told you in the opening pages of this book that many men are ill-equipped to face the ever-raging war of sexual temptations that Satan, the flesh, and the world are waging against their souls.

As every man knows, the daily onslaughts we face predominantly assail the battlefield of our minds. It's on this very ground that we will either surrender defeated or triumph victorious. The outcome will be determined by whether we chose to fight biblically in the ways that we've already explored together.

A big part of our fighting strategy, which involves the mind, must include bringing every thought into captivity to the obedience of Christ (2 Corinthians 10:5), determining to have the mind of Christ (1 Corinthians 2:16), and choosing not to be conformed to this world but instead to be transformed by the renewing of our mind (Romans 12:2). This will require both immersion in truth and a battle plan to summon and appropriate that truth in a preventative, offensive, and defensive way.

When a barrage of sexual temptations inundates a man—usually in the form of unclean thoughts—if his mind is not proactively and deliberately prepared ahead of time, he will be rendered defenseless—with no shield in hand. By the same token, if he has no robust scriptural truth to draw on, he will find himself with no offensive power—with no sword in hand. And having neither shield nor sword, the man will deal with constant assaults because, as we discovered early on in this book, having good defensive and offensive capabilities is essential for preventative preparedness, which will often block attacks from happening in the first place.

In order to arm us with both shield and sword and to make our defensive and offensive capabilities so robust that our enemies would typically be dissuaded from even attacking us, I want to set forth six powerful truths for us to deeply understand, diligently internalize, and daily meditate on. I have designed these points to be both memorable and mentally accessible, especially in the heat of battle.

I formulated these principles quite a while ago, and after memorizing the key word and alliterative sentence associated with each one—in the same order in which they'll appear in this book—I've gotten in the habit of regularly recounting them to myself, contemplating them, and praying through them. The results have been personally transformational, and I've found myself noticeably strengthened and empowered to walk in victory when I've been tempted to give in to lust.

While you'll notice that I've included detailed content in connection with each principle, this shouldn't be intimidating to you. After developing the habit of meditating on these truths, you'll come to realize that, in a matter of seconds, you can unleash in your life the power they contain. Each one of the six principles will flash through your mind in rapid succession when you recall them in a moment of temptation. It will take some time up front, but the long-lasting benefits will be well worth it. This is not to say that you can't maintain a practice of spending a total of five minutes or so every day (or longer if you so desire) meditating on all six principles. That can be a very helpful practice. But you'll notice with time that after you have engrained these biblical truths in your heart and mind, they will become an instant help to you.

Ain't No Chance

From the time I was a little boy and long before I had become a Christian, I was in awe of God's creation. The vastness of space, the order in the cosmos, the intricate design across the animal kingdom, and the breathtaking complexity and ingenuity etched in the human body should be enough to hold spellbound even the least perceptive person. God's fingerprints are all over His creative works of art that fill up the universe. And while men may claim that everything is the by-product of random chance, the book of Romans emphatically declares that everyone knows God exists and that He's made this apparent through the things He has created: "The wrath of God is revealed from heaven against all ungodliness and unrighteousness of men, who suppress the truth in unrighteousness, because what may be known of God is manifest in them, for God has shown it to them. For since the creation of the world His invisible attributes are clearly seen, being understood by the things that are made, even His eternal power and Godhead, so that they are without excuse" (Romans 1:18–20).

After coming to Christ, my eyes were opened even more to the marvels of everything that God had spoken into existence. There was now a personal element connected to it—my Father fashioned it all. *My Father!* This blew my mind and put my appreciation for the Lord's handiwork on steroids. As a new believer in high school, my newfound zeal exploded through the words I penned in this poem titled "Who Can Tell Me?":

"Who can tell me where I came from?"
The little boy would ask.
His question was a good one,
Yet he faced a trying task.

Each man had different answers,
As he was soon to learn.
This brought him great confusion,
And it caused a deep concern.

He first went to his schoolmates,
And they spoke with one another.
"I know," said the brightest one,
"You came from your mother."

Now this had satisfied him,
Yet only for a time.
For as he grew, year by year,
His thoughts began to climb.

He then looked all around him
At all that he could see.
And his mind began to wonder
How it all had come to be.

He thought about the universe,
The span of outer space,
And every star and planet
That exists in every place.

He thought about the rounded Earth,
Its tilt and its rotation,
And all the seasons that occur
In yearly circulation.

He thought about the darkness,
And he thought about the light.
He thought about the sun and moon
That rule the day and night.

He thought of all the creatures
Of the land and sea and skies,
Of all the different species
And their variance in size.

He thought of all the plants and trees
And all that each provides,

Each growing from a tiny seed
With roots the soil hides.

He then looked at humanity,
The sea of different faces,
Varied tongues and characters
From many distant places.

He thought of mortal bodies
With features so profound
And the sense of taste and touch
And smell and sight and sound.

He thought of reproduction
And the miracle of birth.
He thought of human life itself
And all that it is worth.

He then considered human will:
Both the weak and strong.
He thought about the conscience
That discerns the right from wrong.

He thought about emotions
And feelings that arise.
He thought about the love and hate
And tears that flow from eyes.

He thought about the anger
And the joy that's all around.
He thought about the happiness
And sadness that is found.

And filled with curiosity,
This boy would daily strive
In hopeful expectation
That his answer would arrive.

He spoke with scientific men
Who claimed his question solved.
They told him of a great Big Bang,
That all things had evolved.

He then spoke with philosophers—
Heard some of them insist
That there's no true reality
And we do not exist.

He spoke with many people
From different groups and sects
And heard the vast opinions
Of various intellects.

Now baffled by confusion,
A very troubled youth;
Unable to discern
What is error, what is truth.

He almost gave up looking,
But he took a second look.
And very unexpectedly
He found a special Book.

As he gazed upon the first page,
He knew his search was done.
His questions all were answered
In Genesis chapter one.

With a nod of understanding,
He smiled, so elated.
For now he surely knew—
"In the beginning God created…"

The thing that makes sexual sin exceedingly sinful is that instead
of using the evident wonders of God's creation found in the human body
as wellsprings with which to worship Him, we tragically use them as

weapons with which to wound Him. And in the process, we also end up wounding others and ourselves. We need to learn to pause when we're tempted to lust in our hearts or to engage in any sort of sexual sin and, instead, to meditate carefully on the three marvels of the masterfully crafted human body that we use most prominently in that sinful process. I'm talking about vision, cognition, and coition.

Vision

The human eye has been called the window of the soul. It's the gateway to our brain and the initial instrument used to trigger the process of lust in us. To me, vision has always been one of the most worship-inducing features of the human body.

Scientists tell us that eyes consist of more than two million working parts and typically process over thirty-six thousand pieces of information every hour.[1] The human eyes can detect over ten million color hues, and they are protected by lids that blink an average of 5.2 million times per year.[2] Each eye has 137 million light-sensitive cells, with focusing muscles that move an estimated one hundred thousand times per day.[3] Eyes have supersensitive, built-in light meters, wide-angle lenses, immediate automatic focusing mechanisms, and full-color instantaneous reproduction capabilities.

While professional photographers and videographers are far more familiar with the technologically advanced elements of modern cameras, even the average person can agree that the human eye is infinitely more sophisticated than the most sophisticated camera, which its inventors patterned after the eye to begin with.

Cognition

Though it's evident that our eyes are the gateway to allowing lustful images into our mind, our brain is the instrument through which those images are cognitively processed. Its three pounds of squishy gray and white matter contain nearly one hundred billion neurons, or microscopic nerve cells. Each neuron forms connections to other neurons, which in

1   Dr. Russel Lazarus, "How Does the Eye Work?" Optometrists Network, October 11, 2020, https://www.optometrists.org.

2   Luke Ward, "20 Amazing Eye Facts," The Fact Site, May 11, 2020, https://www.thefactsite.com.

3   "Evidence from Anatomy," Creation Facts, September 13, 2009, http://www.creation-facts.org.

turn could lead to trillions of connections. A piece of brain tissue the size of a grain of sand contains one hundred thousand neurons and one billion synapses. When a neuron is stimulated, it generates an electrical impulse that travels from cell to cell at a speed of 268 miles per hour.[4]

What's more, John Barnett shared, "[The brain] contains many times more nerve lines than all the telephone lines in the world put together. The electrical signals from 200,000 living thermometer cells, a half-million pressure-sensing cells, and 3 or 4 million pain-sensing cells are all routed to the brain, plus the signals from the eyes…, the ears, nose, and taste buds…The brain sorts, stores and acts upon these myriad impulses."[5]

Serving as a biological hard drive that runs cerebral software, the brain operates as the control center for the entire body, providing us with the capacity for thinking, reasoning, emoting, memorizing, verbalizing, recalling, imagining, and creating. All the while, it autonomously controls and regulates all pulmonary, cardiovascular, pituitary, and digestive functions without our conscious participation.

Researchers have rightly said that "the brain is the last and grandest biological frontier, the most complex thing we have yet discovered in our universe."[6] While there are claims that supercomputers can and will continue to exceed the human brain's computing speed and capabilities and that artificial intelligence will eventually surpass human intelligence, don't ever forget that these things are the by-products of the brain's infinitely advanced brilliance and ingenuity and that these technological inventions will never even come close to exceeding the human brain's indomitable superiority in any real way.

Richard Butchko, a retired professor of sociology and psychology, when writing about Fugako—the fastest supercomputer in the world at the time, located in Japan—highlighted the fact that Fugako has 7.3 million cores and 415.5 petaflops (which is an incredibly fast calculating speed). Without getting too technical, we can just say that

---

4   Deane Alban, "72 Amazing Human Brain Facts (Based on the Latest Science)," Be Brain Fit, last updated September 21, 2022, https://bebrainfit.com.

5   John Barnett, *Discipline Yourself for Godliness: The Power of a Word Filled Life* (Tulsa, OK: Mullerhaus Publishing, 2007), 417.

6   James D. Watson, foreword to *Discovering the Brain*, by Sandra Ackerman (Washington, DC: National Academies Press, 1992), https://www.ncbi.nlm.nih.gov.

Butchko summed things up by giving some rough figures to compare Fugako's speed and the speed of the human brain in conducting a specific computation.

> A rough calculation would be that if it took a person, working at a rate of, say, 5-seconds to do 1 floating-point operation on a hand calculator, it would take a human with a hand-calculator working at 24/7/365, 32 million years to equal what the Fugaku could do in one second.[7]

Butchko went on to make this ingenious statement:

> Comparisons between the operation of the human brain and computers are difficult to make and the legitimacy of any comparisons can be argued endlessly. Besides comparing hardware and "software," results—output, in terms of the computer, behavior in terms of the human—is another way to compare.
>
> The awesome power and speed of the Fugaku is not to be denied. Yet, it cannot get up from an easy chair, go to the refrigerator, browse for something to eat, decide to snap open a cold one, throw some cheese and tortilla chips into the microwave, sit back in the easy chair, watch a comedy show on television, have a good laugh, read a novel and mentally experience being on a pirate ship in the Caribbean in the 1700s, or cry over the injury of a puppy. A human can cry, laugh, love, experience orgasms, feel empathy, taste food, put him or herself in someone else's shoes, be conscious, experience music, imagine other times and places, and experience wonder, awe, fear, disgust, and excitement… The human brain does this with an energy consumption equivalent to a 20-watt light bulb whereas what the Fugaku does is much, much less and what it does requires millions of watts of energy. Now that's some astounding computing.

---

7   Richard Butchko, answer to "Are Computers Faster Than the Human Brain," Quora, last updated August 23, 2023, https://www.quora.com.

The combination of computer hardware and software that would be necessary to accomplish what a human infant does…in the space of any random five-minute segment of time on any typical day, would make comparing the Fugaku massively parallel supercomputer to the human brain like comparing a paper airplane to a SpaceX Starship.[8]

And what a wonder that the brain, in combination with the immaterial mind and interconnected with the eternal soul, bears witness to the fact that man was made in the divine image of the infinite God who fashioned him.

Whenever you're tempted to lust—whether it's through looking at pornography, staring at a woman who happens to be in front of you, or letting your mind fixate on salacious mental images—don't ever forget the cognitive miracle required to make lustful imaginings even possible.

Coition

Perhaps you're thinking, *Why did you call this section "Coition"? And what in the world is it anyway?* Good questions. Well, things that rhyme are easier to remember, and so it goes well with "Vision" and "Cognition." But the definition also happens to fit perfectly with the important point that I want to cover.

As a word that is synonymous with *coitus, coition* means…drumroll, please…sexual intercourse. Earth-shattering, right? Not really. It's quite simple, actually. But what is extremely earth-shattering and far from simple are the elaborate inner workings of sexual intercourse.

One of the biggest tragedies surrounding sex is that most people don't pause long enough to consider the mechanical marvel that this poetic work of art really is. Many indulge in it thoughtlessly—like instinct-driven animals—fulfilling what they perceive as an uncontrollable urge, never pondering its miraculous features and its multifaceted dimensions. How sad that something so beautiful can be twisted into something so meaningless and, often, so perverted and debased.

Let me just get candid with you and ask how in the world anyone could honestly believe that male and female genitalia were fashioned through a long and blind process of evolution. Not to mention the fact that this process had to be replicated in every sexually reproducing species in existence. Never mind that these species could not reproduce until their corresponding sexual organs were fully formed, functional, and capable of leading to viable conception. Anyone who believes that human sex organs evolved randomly is completely ignorant about the complex nature of these organs and their operations, or because they are so bent on being autonomous from God, they have obstinately marched themselves into willful ignorance.

From attraction to desire to arousal to anatomical compatibility to unspeakable ecstasy experienced through orgasmic pleasure, sex is no coincidence. And if those things alone don't enthrall you, think about the ultimate miraculous outcome of sexual intimacy: procreation. Two separate individuals engaging in what is supposed to be a loving, intensely bonding, and deeply satisfying act unite to produce, through their sublime oneness, a new human life that contains bits of them both.

When exploring reproduction, we come across terms like *ovulation, fertilization,* and *implantation.* It's easy to just skim over them and not genuinely grasp the intricacies of these stunning processes.

Without ovulation, it's impossible for a woman to conceive. This is because there would be no egg present for the man to fertilize. From the millions of follicles in a woman's ovaries to the growth and development of those follicles through the diffusion of special hormones during menstruation to the stimulation of those follicles through the luteinizing hormone—all these elements must be present, and each of these steps must work flawlessly in order for an egg to be released and have a successful trek toward the uterine cavity.

As sexual intimacy reaches its climax, hundreds of millions of sperm cells from the man release and begin their voyage toward the awaiting egg. The mission? Fertilization. But the sperm must survive the treacherous journey to the fallopian tube as they cross the harsh and foreboding terrain of the cervix and uterus. Very few make it. And within this twenty-four-hour period before the egg dies and can no longer be fertilized, one sperm out of the massive throng must be the first to penetrate the egg's outer shell—the zona pellucida. Once the winner claims his prize, the outer shell of the egg instantly changes and blocks the entry of any other sperm cells.

After the first cell splits, an explosion of cell division and growth activity triggers inside the zygote, and from there the cells continue to multiply by a factor of two, transforming into about fifty to one hundred cells over the next four to six days. After the fertilized embryo descends the fallopian tube and makes its way into the uterus, it bursts forth from its encasement and attaches to the endometrium of the uterus. At this point, implantation takes place, connecting baby and mother in a transforming, biological bond.[9]

Now begins the acceleration of the magical development process as the precious child develops in accordance with the information encoded in their inherited DNA. Scientists tell us that the human genome, the set of chromosomes that contain the baby's complete genetic information, is made up of 3.2 billion sets of genetic "letters." And that "in order to list all those letters, a person would have to type 60 words per minute, 8 hours a day, for about 50 years!"[10] We know that DNA from just one of our cells would stretch out to six feet in length if each strand were uncoiled and they were placed end to end. If this were done for all our DNA, the strand would end up being sixty-seven billion miles long. That's the same distance as 150,000 round trips to the moon.[11]

That incredible DNA information determines everything about the baby developing in the womb—their height; the size and shape of their hands, feet, nose, and ears; the nuances of their facial features; their skin, eye, and hair color; the cadence of their voice; their temperament; their personality; the acuteness of their senses; and all their physical and mental capabilities.

Think of it! The whole miracle of life that we just pondered is directly linked to this magnificent event called coition—the wonderful gift of sexual intimacy. God designed coition to provide pleasure, strengthen unity, and create life. When we give in to lust, pornography, masturbation, adultery, homosexuality, or any other form of sexual

9 "The Miracles of Conception: Back to the Basics," Rocky Mountain Fertility Center, July 25, 2014, https://www.rockymountainfertility.com.
10 Chelsea Toledo and Kirstie Saltsman, "Genetics by the Numbers," National Institute of General Medical Sciences, June 12, 2012, https://www.nigms.nih.gov.
11 Toledo and Saltsman, "Genetics by the Numbers."

CREATION

immorality, we pervert this beautiful gift and dishonor the gracious God who gave it to us—the God who means for us to use it in accordance with the loving and divine intentions He has for it.

So the next time you're tempted to sin sexually, immediately think, *Creation*, and then reflect on the intricate, breathtaking, and mind-blowing details associated with vision, cognition, and coition. Finally, decide to use the astounding faculties and features that God has placed in your body as wellsprings or sources through which to express your awe of Him and honor Him instead of using them as instruments through which to sinfully wound Him, yourself, and others. And say to yourself, *Creation: wield wonders as wellsprings for worship, not weapons for wounding.*

The exploration of creation whisks us to the most sacred and sobering spot in the universe, the foot of the cross.

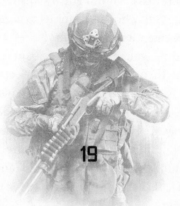

19

CROSS

STOP SPITTING AND STOMPING
ON SUCH A SACRED SYMBOL

Cross-Purposes

We wear it around our necks, dangle it from our ears, tattoo it onto our bodies, and hoist it atop our church steeples. We carve replicas, paint pictures, and mold sculptures of it. And our hearts well up with solemn emotions when we raise our voices and sing about it. But do we carry it? Do we crucify ourselves on it? And do we understand the incalculable price that our Savior paid when He allowed wicked men to impale Him on it—for us—for wretched sinners to whom He owed nothing but wrath and judgment?

I stared at it as it hung in our church chapel Sunday after Sunday. It certainly commanded my respect and attention but in a very compartmentalized way. I guess in the same compartmentalized way that it commanded the respect and attention of the man who had it tattooed on his forearm and then afterward used that same forearm to clothesline someone in a selfish fit of rage. Have you ever listened to a belligerent man spew vile vulgarities and obscenities with a crucifix hanging just inches beneath his lips? And what of the stories you've heard about supposed ministers of the cross committing serial adultery with their congregants and molesting the children in their flock?

Whether men give lip service to how much they value the cross and yet spurn it by living in opposition to all that it represents or whether they outright disdain it and viciously revile it, Scripture is clear on the reasons for their rejection. We're told in 1 Corinthians 1:18: "The message of the cross is foolishness to those who are perishing."

Hypocrites and heathens alike don't really grasp the message of the cross. In fact, it's more than just bewildering to them. The cross, in their estimation and judging by their actions, whether consciously or subconsciously, is a symbol of utter folly, and by extension, it is completely worthless and useless to them.

As R. C. Sproul powerfully stated, the cross is far from worthless and useless to the one who ordained it: "The sweetest fragrance, the most beautiful aroma that God has ever detected emanating from this planet, was the aroma of the perfect sacrifice of Jesus that was offered once and for all on the cross."[1]

Cross-Examination

As we turn now to examine the rest of 1 Corinthians 1:18, we discover that it goes on to say, "To us who are being saved it is the power of God." To the true believer, the cross is not a fashion accessory. It's not a good luck charm or an emblem that wards off evil spirits. It's far more than a religious symbol to be lauded and revered. The cross is everything to a Christian. It's the very source of their rescue, their redemption, their regeneration. It's God's power unveiled and unleashed toward them in extravagant and overabundant love—a love that far exceeds comprehension: "That you, being rooted and grounded in love, may be able to comprehend with all the saints what is the width and length and depth and height—to know the love of Christ which passes knowledge; that you may be filled with all the fullness of God" (Ephesians 3:17–19).

When you examine the details of your battle against sexual sin, do you find that it's fueled by the power of the cross? In other words, is your resistance a cross-centered one? How often does your mind cast its

---

1   R. C. Sproul, *The Purpose of God: An Exposition of Ephesians* (Fearn, Ross-shire, UK: Christian Focus Publications, 1994), 121.

gaze on the cross and all that it signifies when the devil, the flesh, and the world are all raging against you and pulling you toward the brink of mutiny against the God whom you claim to love above all else? Along with your remembering the glories of God's creation by meditating on the amazing realities we explored when we looked at the first C (creation), the cross (which is represented by the second C) should become a daily focus in your life. It must be the instrument that conquers you and the one through which you conquer sexual sin.

Crossing Yourself

In the opening chapter of his epistle to the Philippians, Paul challenged his readers to let their conduct be "worthy of the gospel of Christ" (1:27). As 1 Corinthians 15 tells us, the heart of the gospel is the death, burial, and resurrection of our Savior. The cross, obviously being the instrument of Jesus' substitutionary death for His people, is the necessary precursor of His burial and resurrection; it's the gateway to the fullness of the gospel's splendors. Here we find Paul employing *worthy* to describe how Christians should walk in connection with the components of the gospel, which, again, chronologically begin with the cross.

The word *worthy* carries with it the idea of a perfectly balanced scale, where a particular object on one side fully matches the weight of a separate object placed on the other side. The thrust of what Paul was saying is that the believer should live in such a way that their actions match the weighty value of the gospel. The practical outworking of this surrender is that the man of God, in the heat of sexual temptation, turns his gaze toward the cross and considers its horror, its solemnity, its beauty, its eternal significance, its redeeming power, and its transformational impact. Then, in an act of total surrender, he willingly rejects the temptation to surrender to sexual sin and instead chooses to walk in the self-control that demonstrates how much he truly values the pricelessness of the cross.

Why didn't God send an angel or a prophet or even fashion an altogether new being of sorts to save us from ourselves? It's because only an infinite Being could bear the infinite punishment that man deserved for the infinite wickedness of his sin. Think of it: Christ chose to leave the splendors of His eternal kingdom, don a robe of flesh, and suffer on a cruel cross at the hands of His own creation. He not only endured the blasphemies that issued forth from the very vocal cords, tongues, and lips He had crafted, but He even allowed Himself to be crucified on a wooden beam that came from a tree that His own hand had fashioned, with spikes that were forged from the very iron He created. And He did it all willingly.

What are the ramifications associated with the cross? What should we be pondering as we discipline ourselves to regularly meditate on it? While we know that the cross was the instrument through which Jesus secured our salvation, what are some of the other effects that it should have on us in the course of our journey toward heaven?

As God became one of us so that He could save us *from* Himself (meaning from His just wrath) and *for* Himself, Scripture tells us that "He died for all, that those who live should live no longer for themselves, but for Him who died for them and rose again" (2 Corinthians 5:15). It's paramount that we recognize the import of this truth. This is accentuated even more when we remember that Scripture directly connects the work of the cross to our call to walk in sexual purity: "Flee sexual immorality. Every sin that a man does is outside the body, but he who commits sexual immorality sins against his own body. Or do you not know that your body is the temple of the Holy Spirit who is in you, whom you have from God, and you are not your own? For you were bought at a price; therefore glorify God in your body and in your spirit, which are God's" (1 Corinthians 6:18–20).

CrossFit

While the cross secures our eternal destiny, it also provides an avenue for our liberation from the influences and control of this godless world: "Our Lord Jesus Christ...gave Himself for our sins, that He might deliver us from this present evil age, according to the will of our God and Father" (Galatians 1:3–4).

Paul likewise highlighted the very practical purposes of God's saving grace, made available to God's children through the death of Christ for them on the cross:

> The grace of God that brings salvation has appeared to all men, teaching us that, denying ungodliness and worldly lusts, we should live soberly, righteously, and godly in the present age, looking for the blessed hope and glorious appearing of our great God and Savior Jesus Christ, who gave Himself for us, that He might redeem us from every lawless deed and purify for Himself His own special people, zealous for good works.
>
> Speak these things, exhort, and rebuke with all authority. Let no one despise you. (Titus 2:11–15)

This immeasurable, cross-centered grace diffuses itself through a teaching ministry that instructs the objects of its transforming power to deny every form of ungodliness and the lure of the world's toxic lust. The very reason for which Christ "gave Himself for us" as a sacrifice on that cruel Roman gibbet was to buy us out of bondage to the lawless ways of our darkened hearts. His intent is to purify us as His own "special" people—those who are set apart, distinct from this world, and, therefore, wholly consecrated unto Him—a type of people who cast aside passivity and complacency and who burn with a passionate zeal to cast off evil works and instead fulfill good works of righteousness unto His glory.

This becomes clearer as we read Paul's famous words to the Galatians: "I have been crucified with Christ; it is no longer I who live, but Christ lives in me; and the life which I now live in the flesh I live by faith in the Son of God, who loved me and gave Himself for me" (Galatians 2:20).

The cross is a reminder to us that we are called to identify with our Savior's crucifixion by giving up our lives as He gave up His for us and, in turn, yielding to Christ living in us and through us. This harkens back to the words of Jesus when He articulated the cost of discipleship: "Jesus said to His disciples, 'If anyone desires to come after Me, let him deny himself, and take up his cross, and follow Me'" (Matthew 16:24).

John MacArthur's words effectively capture the essence of Christ's call to the crucified life: "Here is why all the central truths of the gospel focus on the cross: It reveals how heinous our sin is. It shows the intensity of God's wrath against sin. It reveals the great love of God in paying such a high price for redemption. But it also serves as a fitting metaphor for the cost of following Christ. Jesus himself spoke repeatedly of the cross in those terms."[2]

Those who do take up their cross of self-denial and follow in Jesus' footsteps will eventually be able to wholeheartedly echo the words of the faithful apostle Paul, who resolutely exclaimed, "God forbid that I should boast except in the cross of our Lord Jesus Christ, by whom the world has been crucified to me, and I to the world" (Galatians 6:14).

While we are speaking about metaphorical crucifixion, the apostle Andrew was crucified in the most literal way imaginable. Read these words that he was said to have uttered as he headed toward his cross: "Oh, cross most welcome and longed for! With a willing mind, joyfully and desirously, I come to you, being a scholar of Him which did hang on you, because I have always been your lover and yearn to embrace you."[3] May we follow in his footsteps as we daily bear our cross of self-denial and surrender to Christ.

Cross-Eyed

You'll find no greater deterrent to surrendering to sexual sin than meditating on the cross in a moment of temptation. Envisioning the torture and torment that Christ endured to save you from sin will rescue you from the perilous brink of delusion and folly.

When you imagine the spectacle of the cross and peer through your mind's eye at the visage of the God-man, the one who was marred beyond recognition, do you see His battered, bruised, and mangled body? Can your imagination focus on His noble head adorned with a crown of thorns and His lacerated arms dripping with blood and extended in love for you? Can you make out the details of His nail-pierced hands, the same ones that touched lepers, healed blind eyes, and washed His disciples' filthy feet?

It's within the atmosphere of this sober contemplation that you must will yourself into understanding the severity of capitulating to sexual temptations as you stand in the shadow of the cross—the very

---

2   John MacArthur, *Successful Christian Parenting: Raising Your Child with Care, Compassion, and Common Sense* (Nashville, TN: Thomas Nelson, 1998), 62.

3   Allyson Holland, "Who Were the 12 Disciples and What Should We Know about Them?" Crosswalk, January 27, 2020, https://www.crosswalk.com.

cross that held Him who so lovingly endured such unspeakable shame and torment for you.

Can you, with one eye on the cross, turn your other eye toward sexually perverse images that stir lust within you? Can you, with one hand raised in praise to God for the cross, simultaneously use the other hand to lewdly touch yourself? Can you, with your body crucified on the cross with Christ, allow it to engage in sexual immorality with another?

If you brazenly do these things, then understand that you are, in essence, spitting on the cross as though it were worthless, trampling it beneath your feet as though it were trash, and declaring with your actions that it means nothing whatsoever to you. And you *must* think this way. Allow these sobering thoughts to snap you back into reality and provoke you to flee the folly of iniquity as you pursue the pathway of righteousness for the glory of the one who is worth it. When you're tempted to betray the cross and the Savior, who hung on it, say to yourself, *Cross: stop spitting and stomping on such a sacred symbol.*

Having explored creation and cross, we will now move on to examine crisis in the next chapter.

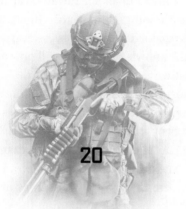

20

CRISIS

CONSIDER THE CATASTROPHIC
CONSEQUENCES OF COMPROMISE

Awake or Leave a Wake of Destruction

Collins *Dictionary* aptly defines the word *crisis* as "a situation in which something or someone is affected by one or more very serious problems." The real issue at hand is not that crises are a reality that we're all susceptible to experiencing, as this clearly comes with the territory when living in a fallen, broken, and sin-saturated world. The danger is that Christians often ignore the serious ramifications that come with self-inflicted crises and become deceived into thinking that they are not likely to make the sorts of mistakes that will bring crises into their lives. This triggers complacency at its worst and puts the Christian at risk of stumbling into one catastrophic crisis after another.

When blinded by the lure of sexual sin, it's easy to suppress in our minds the reality of its consequences. As hormones rage and our bodies flood with a surge of dopamine, nitrogen oxide, and noradrenaline, we can easily lose all sense of reality and get swallowed up in a state of euphoric insanity.[1] But all sin-fueled escapades come with loads of built-in regret on the other side of the climax. Once the tension is released and we've regained our scruples, we are left with that cold, hollow feeling and the knowledge that we will now begin the devastating work of reaping what we've sown. Enter crisis.

There is no shortage of crisis-filled examples associated with sexual immorality—whether from our own lives, the lives of people we know personally, or the lives of others we've heard about. The wise man makes it his daily habit to pause and reflect on such examples, to learn from them, and to take whatever steps necessary to avoid repeating them.

A well-known friend of mine who serves in the leadership of a high-profile ministry keeps a list containing the names of pastors and Christian leaders who have fallen into sexual immorality. The sad fact is that the list is quite long, and tragically, it keeps getting longer with each passing year. Having seen that this practice serves my friend well, I've created my own list of those whom I've known or have heard about who have shipwrecked their lives and the lives of many others because they chose to violate sexual integrity and not walk in self-control. As my mind scrolls through the faces of these men, I'm sadly reminded of the trail of destruction that they have left in their wake. I recall the broken marriages, the devastated and embittered children, the ravaged ministries, and the demolished churches with wounded, disillusioned, and distraught congregants. Let's also not forget the countless unbelievers who had some semblance of respect toward those fallen, professing Christians and before whose eyes the testimony of the gospel was marred. And, of course, we have to remember the enemies of the faith and recall the prophet Nathan's words to King David after he committed adultery with Bathsheba, had her husband Uriah murdered, and hid his sin: "By this deed you have given great occasion to the enemies of the LORD to blaspheme" (2 Samuel 12:14).

And while these are the more obvious crisis situations that can result from sexual sin, there are many other crippling crises that have the power to radically weaken and derail men. Society often minimizes these types of crises because the world does not value the concepts associated

---

1   Michelle Clarke, "What's Going On with Hormones and Neurotransmitters during Sex," Atlas Blog, June 25, 2023, https://atlasbiomed.com.

with them. I'm talking about conscience, moral authority, leadership capacity, witness, and joy.

Crisis of Conscience: The One Con You Don't Want to Become an Ex

The sins of my youth ravaged my life in more ways than I care to recount. But my conscience took the brunt of the decimating blows that I had inflicted on myself. Anytime I ventured into newer areas of sin, I distinctly felt its amplified twinges. But the more I persisted in my waywardness, the more desensitized my conscience became. Eventually, while I could still hear its muffled screams, they slowly grew fainter and more distant. And in rare moments when my conscience managed to somehow sneak in a discernible plea for restraint, I would immediately drown it out by intensifying the deafening noise of my rebellious sin.

All that changed, however, on the night that Christ invaded my life and transformed me. He gave me a new heart, a new mind, a new hunger for righteousness, and then He topped it all off with a hypersensitive conscience. Anytime I even thought about sinning, I was blinded by its brightly flashing warning lights and rattled by its ear-splitting sirens. But as time went on in my fledgling faith, I found myself, on occasion, ignoring the voice of my conscience in certain areas. In place of desensitization, I felt a deep sense of grief that was like a rain cloud hovering over me wherever I went. I had no peace in my soul and was constantly conflicted as I wrestled with my troubled and tormented conscience. As a Christian who was indwelt by the Spirit of God, I came to experience firsthand the significance of the old adage "There's no softer pillow than a clear conscience."

Can you relate to this? Perhaps when you first were saved, you immediately yielded to the convictions of your conscience when it came to lust. You willed yourself into diverting your eyes from women's bodies and from allowing your imagination to venture into perverse territory. But over time, you gave in to the pull. Then, before you knew it, the occasional glances, which were separated by intervals of self-control, became habitual. This then led you to periodically look at pornography and masturbate. And over time, even these activities became commonplace and regular occurrences in your life.

Let me ask you how your conscience fared during that season of your life. Did you have peace? Did you find yourself hungering for God's Word? Were you excited about sitting through convicting sermons? Were you engaging in deep fellowship, in open accountability, and in zealous evangelism? Perhaps you are currently in that season of life. Then ask yourself those same questions about your current predicament. I think I know the answers, and so do you. Your crisis of conscience makes it impossible to fully enter into those sorts of things with any real measure of freedom and excitement. When we're not walking uprightly, we typically steer clear of the light. Holy activities are uncomfortable, and they awaken in our conscience those feelings of guilt and conviction that we're seeking to suppress.

Crisis of Moral Authority: When Silence Isn't Golden

I'm sure you've seen your fair share of corny scenes in B movies where one character is standing next to someone who is being reprimanded for something shameful that they've done. The camera then zooms in on the bystander's face as they swallow hard and rapidly shift their eyes back and forth while beads of sweat form on their brow. The overdramatized acting is clearly meant to convey that they're guilty of the same thing that the person next to them is being rebuked for. While people in the real world may sometimes be better actors than on-screen professionals, we all know how much we want to avoid discussing something that may pull the veil back from our own embarrassing sins.

When we surrender to the whims of sexual temptations, we will face repercussions that are far worse than embarrassment. Those whom we care about may be indulging in the very same sins, but we will be muzzled and stripped of our moral authority to speak. Can you imagine this happening with your brother, son, dad, nephew, cousin, or close friend? You discover that he is ensnared in the clutches of sexual immorality. You know that he respects you enough to listen to your counsel and input, but you realize that it would be the height of hypocrisy to exhort him to repent of something that you yourself are habitually engaging in.

The disastrous consequences associated with this one crisis alone should be enough to strike sobriety into the heart of any man who has even the slightest semblance of care for the other men in his life. Think of the repercussions that can result from silence over a matter this serious and consider that those to whom you've pledged your life and love and loyalty will be the ones who experience these devastating repercussions. Are they not worth your sacrifice and self-denial of fleeting, unlawful, and destructive pleasures?

If you are currently living in sexual sin and are not struck with an urgency to repent in light of what you just read, then you should be extremely concerned about the state of your soul. In other words, do what's right by crying out to God for forgiveness and help anyway—even if you don't feel like it. He stands ready and willing to be the source of your rescue.

Crisis of Leadership Capacity: No Footsteps to Follow In

While the crisis of losing the moral authority to speak up about destructive sins in the lives of those we treasure is devastating, there is yet another crucial area where we can find ourselves tragically weakened. I'm talking about leadership.

The large salaries that CEOs of major corporations receive often amaze people. They wonder why someone would get paid so much money to spend half their week on the golf course and the other half enjoying expensive lunches and dinners in swanky restaurants—and perhaps occasionally signing a few papers, sitting in some meetings (with tasty snacks), and giving people orders to carry out. Not to mention the constant zipping around on private jets to exotic locations around the globe.

While that description might be a bit overglamorized, it's not too far off the mark, at least from a surface-level perspective. This is especially true when contrasted with the labor-intensive work that most employees of major corporations do. And we can't forget their astronomically low wages by comparison.

However, those who have an understanding of how the real world works are well aware that without the CEO, major corporations would not exist in the first place, nor would they continue to grow, thrive, and function effectively. This speaks to the enormous influence of good leadership. The same goes for the leadership of a nation. Is it any wonder that when one country invades another, the top priority is usually to capture or assassinate the head of state? A leadership vacuum immediately destabilizes the government and demoralizes the population. A good leader, by the sheer power of his presence, example, words, and actions, can inspire, encourage, enthuse, embolden, and activate others in extraordinary ways. That's why the CEO—who bears great responsibility, endures enormous stress, and generates massive impact—gets the big bucks.

Knowing how powerful and important upstanding leadership is, corporations typically have a "good behavior" clause in their CEO's contract that gives the board of directors the right to dismiss him or her for unethical or immoral conduct. The same holds true for high-ranking government officials and even Supreme Court justices, who are appointed for life. In fact, the United States Constitution enshrines this standard for those who will serve on the bench of the highest court in the land: "The judicial Power of the United States, shall be vested in one supreme Court, and in such inferior Courts as the Congress may from time to time ordain and establish. The Judges, both of the supreme and inferior Courts, shall hold their Offices during good behaviour" (Article III, Section 1). Character matters, and everyone knows that institutions can crumble at every level if the person at the top is not functioning to the fullest of their leadership capacity.

While no one may officially remove you from the various relational leadership roles you hold in the lives of others, you essentially remove yourself when you squelch your ability to exert influence because of secret or public sexual sin. This is because living in rebellion against God kills your integrity, your vision, your passion, and your voice. And without these elements, you won't want to lead anyone, and no one will want to follow you.

Crisis of Witness: A Bunch of Hypocrites

I've already highlighted evangelism as one of the key activities that enable us to involve ourselves in the things that God's Spirit is involved in. We discovered that evangelism helps strengthen us to walk in (or be controlled by) the Spirit of God. However, it's important that we grasp the seriousness of the crisis that results when our ability to be effective witnesses for Christ is diminished.

I want to encourage you to think back to all the times when you've observed unbelievers complain about Christians. What is one of the foremost accusations you've heard them level against those who claim to be disciples of Christ? It goes something like this: "Christians are a bunch of hypocrites. There's this guy at work who says he's a Christian, but he's always cussing up a storm, slacking off on the jobsite, and getting hammered at parties on the weekend." Does that sound familiar? Or how about this one? "I hired this guy to remodel my house. I thought he would be trustworthy and have some integrity because he had a Christian fish on his website. But he turned out to be a big scam artist and did a shoddy job."

Hypocrisy doesn't just hinder our witness when others see our sin on display. It hinders our witness even when our sin is secret. This is because when we are giving ourselves over to such things as sexual immorality, the last thing we want to do is proclaim the gospel to others. So persisting in sin doesn't just hinder our witness; it also often keeps us from witnessing altogether. When we don't walk in a manner worthy of the gospel, we run as far away as we can from proclaiming that gospel. How tragic that we exchange the greatest honor that man has ever known for something so temporal, fading, and dishonoring to God's call on our lives as His representatives.

When I think of all that the apostle Paul endured for the sake of winning souls, I'm deeply convicted. When he was a prisoner in Rome, he penned these words to the believers in Philippi:

> I want you to know, brethren, that the things which happened to me have actually turned out for the furtherance of the gospel, so that it has become evident to the whole palace guard, and to all the rest, that my chains are in Christ; and most of the brethren in the Lord, having become confident by my chains, are much more bold to speak the word without fear.
>
> Some indeed preach Christ even from envy and strife, and some also from goodwill: The former preach Christ from selfish ambition, not sincerely, supposing to add affliction to my chains; but the latter out of love, knowing that I am appointed for the defense of the gospel.

What then? Only that in every way, whether in pretense or in truth, Christ is preached; and in this I rejoice, yes, and will rejoice. (Philippians 1:12–18)

Think of it! Paul seems almost to forget he's a prisoner. He was so consumed with others being touched by the gospel and inspired to proclaim it that he spoke of rejoicing as long as Christ is preached. He said this with full knowledge that some who were preaching Christ with impure motives were actually heaping more affliction on him in the course of his imprisonment.

Is it any wonder that Paul said he endured all things for the sake of the elect so that they may be saved (2 Timothy 2:10), that he became all things to all men in order to save some (1 Corinthians 9:22), and that if he could, he would wish that he were accursed from Christ if it meant that his fellow countrymen would come to know Jesus (Romans 9:3)? Only a man with that sort of heart to be a faithful witness could write the following words: "Now I go bound in the spirit to Jerusalem, not knowing the things that will happen to me there, except that the Holy Spirit testifies in every city, saying that chains and tribulations await me. But none of these things move me; nor do I count my life dear to myself, so that I may finish my race with joy, and the ministry which I received from the Lord Jesus, to testify to the gospel of the grace of God" (Acts 20:22–24).

What a true crisis it is when men give up the power to live such a surrendered and gospel-centered life in exchange for worthless pleasures.

Crisis of Joy: A Waterless Waterfall

Joy is more than just a desirable feeling. It's an animating and empowering element that's available to every regenerated child of God. It's an essential ingredient to the Christian life. Can you imagine living without joy? It would be as pleasurable as listening to an orchestra without instruments, watching a theater production without actors, and having dinner without food. Rainbows need color, sunrises need a sun, waterfalls need water, and for life to be all that God intended it to be for the believer, it must be filled with joy. But how is that possible when there are so many tragedies and so much pain surrounding us? We can find the answer in joy's true definition.

Unlike the transient and conditional nature of happiness, which is directly tied to pleasant emotions and favorable circumstances, joy inherently possesses a much deeper, richer, and more enduring quality. It enables its possessor to smile while they're weeping, sing while they're mourning, and somehow experience an indescribable sense of healing while they're deeply wounded. And though it may seem paradoxical, there's actually a very logical reason behind this phenomenon. It's because real joy is rooted in both a person and a promise—or, more accurately put, a promised person: the Holy Spirit.

As Christians, we're well aware of the fact that we serve a God who is triune in nature. We know, biblically speaking, that He is one divine Being who has always existed as three distinct persons, all coeternal and coequal in essence. While the Trinity is difficult for us to fully grasp and comprehend, it seems that the person within the Godhead who is most challenging for us to connect with and properly understand is the Holy Spirit. You never hear anyone refer to the Father or the Son as "it," but it's quite common for believers to erroneously do this when referring to the Spirit. This gives the impression that we think of the Spirit as more of an impersonal force of sorts rather than the personal deity He really is.

There are multiple passages of Scripture that make it clear that the Holy Spirit is indeed a person and that this person is unquestionably God. The same, of course, holds true for the Father and the Son. And when you have three distinct persons who are all called God yet the Bible makes it clear that there is only one God, you inevitably arrive at the doctrine of the Trinity. There are no portions of Scripture that are more emphatic about the fact that there is only one God than these two in the book of Isaiah:

- "'You are My witnesses,' says the LORD, 'and My servant whom I have chosen, that you may know and believe Me, and understand that I am He. Before Me there was no God formed, nor shall there be after Me'" (Isaiah 43:10).

- "I am the LORD, and there is no other; there is no God besides Me. I will gird you, though you have not known Me, that they may know from the rising of the

sun to its setting that there is none besides Me. I am
the LORD, and there is no other" (Isaiah 45:5–6).

And yet, when Christ gave His disciples the Great Commission, He
spoke clearly of one God, saying they were to be baptized "in the name of
the Father, and of the Son and of the Holy Spirit" (Matthew 28:19).

When it comes to substantiating the personhood and deity of the
Holy Spirit, a very powerful account in the book of Acts does this clearly.
Chapter 5 includes a well-known passage about Ananias and Sapphira,
who lied about how much money they had donated to the church from
a piece of property they had sold. When Peter confronted the couple, he
asked them a very pointed question: "Ananias, why has Satan filled your
heart to lie to the Holy Spirit and keep back part of the price of the land
for yourself?" (v. 3). After saying a few more words, Peter made this very
enlightening statement: "You have not lied to men but to God" (v. 4).
We see here that the apostle confirmed that the Holy Spirit is a person—
since an impersonal force cannot be lied to—and then explicitly confirmed that the Holy Spirit is God.

The Bible contains many more verses that reaffirm the personhood and deity of the Holy Spirit. But relative to His personhood is the
significant fact that He indwells us. We know this because Scripture
makes it clear that each believer is the temple of the Holy Spirit
(1 Corinthians 3:16) and that we are sealed by Him for the day of
redemption (Ephesians 1:13–14).

It's no wonder that God's Word tells us that our thoughts, words,
and actions can grieve the Spirit (4:30). And at the same time, we have a
promise that because the person of the Holy Spirit dwells within us, we
can bear His fruit in our lives (Galatians 5:22–23). Thankfully, we find
that one of the manifestations of the fruit of the Spirit in the life of the
believer is that sweet attribute of joy that we have been exploring.

However, as unconditional as joy is by its very nature and as readily
available as it is to those who house the Spirit of God within them, we
can nonetheless suppress our ability to experience that joy in our lives.
We do this by choosing to walk in the flesh through indulging in sin
and thereby grieving the Holy Spirit. And if the Spirit of God within us
is grieved, how can we possibly experience the joy that comes directly
from Him?

Forfeiting the joy of the Spirit—and thereby diminishing our existence to a joyless meandering through the dark and abysmal labyrinth of life—is the unavoidable outcome of bowing before the cruel god of sexual perversion. And what a true crisis it is to rob ourselves of that joy-filled, sustaining strength that comes from living in harmony with our promised helper (John 14:26). Minimizing the value of the Spirit's joy is a common by-product of our spiritual shortsightedness, but God's Word assures us that joy is an integral part of His kingdom's foundation, "for the kingdom of God is not eating and drinking, but righteousness and peace and joy in the Holy Spirit" (Romans 14:17).

As you contemplate the serious repercussions connected with the element of crisis, I hope that you can see the importance of thriving in the areas associated with it, namely conscience, moral authority, leadership capacity, witness, and joy. If you have previously failed to see this important connection, I pray that your perspective has dramatically shifted. It's crucial that we carefully consider how the crises in connection with the four areas just mentioned—and explored in this chapter—can radically weaken and derail us. As you contemplate all this, I encourage you to regularly say to yourself, *Crisis: consider the catastrophic consequences of compromise.*

Creation, cross, and crisis now lead us to the doorstep of crown.

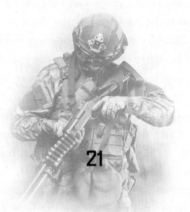

21

CROWN

ENVISION ENDURANCE ENSURING ETERNAL ENRICHMENT

What Would You Do for a Klondike Bar?

I've never been the "What would you do for a Klondike Bar?" kind of a guy. Gold stars in school couldn't motivate me to get my homework done or to behave in class. The "Get a free (and cheesy) duffel bag if you convince your friend to sign up for a gym membership" tactic didn't work on me. And I wasn't one to give the time of day to the annoying "Win a free T-shirt" contests. Worthless wares and rewards were just not a temptation for me. But when I was a teenager and had the opportunity to win a nice television set just for signing people up for newspaper subscriptions, I didn't think twice about accepting the challenge, and I bagged the prize.

I briefly touched on the matter of rewards earlier in this book, but did you know that the Bible is filled with verses that talk about an abundance of rich rewards that God has available for His children? This is perhaps one of the most overlooked truths in Scripture. Could it be the result of confusion on the part of believers? Is it possible that Christians have developed a mental block when it comes to this glorious truth because they've somehow mistaken rewards for a works-based salvation of sorts? You may be surprised to discover that eternal rewards are far more valuable and far more important than you may have imagined.

What's Faith Got to Do with It?

Whenever God's Word specifically underscores something that He wants us to know, we would be very wise to pay close attention to it. This is especially critical when the information is related to one of the Bible's most significant themes—faith. While we know that "the just shall live by faith" (Romans 1:17) and that "faith is the substance of things hoped for, the evidence of things not seen" (Hebrews 11:1), something else about faith strikes at the very heart of the Christian's primary calling in life. Faith, the Bible tells us, is the foundational means by which we can bring pleasure to the heart of God: "Without faith it is impossible to please Him" (Hebrews 11:6).

The Lord is not dazzled by our aspirations, our ambitions, and our accomplishments. He is drawn toward those who demonstrate trust in Him and His Word through faith—the type of humble faith that those mentioned throughout Hebrews 11 exemplified. In the second part of Hebrews 11:6, the author of Hebrews went on to highlight two components that are the basic building blocks for this sort of faith: "He who comes to God must believe that He is, and that He is a rewarder of those who diligently seek Him."

It's obvious that faith's initial step must be an acknowledgment of God's existence. Romans 1 minces no words about the fact that every person knows that God exists because He has revealed this undeniable reality by means of His creation. However, we must deliberately and proactively acknowledge this truth through the vehicle of faith. And the second factor that's interconnected with God-pleasing faith is belief that the Lord rewards those who diligently seek Him.

If this verse caught you by surprise, welcome to my club. While I could understand God revealing truth about rewarding those who diligently seek Him, I would have never expected Him to pair that dynamic with the kind of faith that must accompany those who come to Him.

This has massive implications. The biggest takeaway is that we, as God's people, must believe He will reward those who diligently seek Him. This is a prime truth that God really wants us to deeply grasp and

FIGHT LIKE A MAN

understand. And what a delight that is—both the fact that God wants us to know His heart toward us in this regard and that this is indeed His heart toward us.

If God is telling us that those who diligently seek Him can gain rewards, the natural question to ask is how we should go about seeking the Lord. The specific word that the writer of Hebrews employed for "seek" means "to search for," "to investigate," or "to scrutinize," but it also means "to beg" or "to crave."[1] This type of seeking after God bears the marks of eagerness, urgency, diligence, and determination.

When speaking to the children of Israel through the prophet Jeremiah, God clearly indicated what type of seekers end up truly finding Him: "You will call upon Me and go and pray to Me, and I will listen to you. And you will seek Me and find Me, when you search for Me with all your heart" (Jeremiah 29:12–13). A diligent pursuit of God is rooted and grounded in wholeheartedness. It requires the entirety of one's being— total passion, commitment, dedication, and devotion. Its ultimate demonstration is in total surrender and unconditional obedience. This means that even in the face of life's difficulties, challenges, and intense temptations, along with the struggle, the pain, and even the confusion that might arise at times, we maintain a proactive pursuit of God. And it's this type of diligent and tenacious pursuit of God that He promises to reward.

It must be noted, however, that a passionate pursuit of God is inseparable from a passionate pursuit of bringing Him glory in all things. Mark Hitchcock, in his excellent book *Heavenly Rewards: Living with Eternity in Sight*, drove this point home powerfully with a very enlightening story:

> When the famous pastor H. A. Ironside was a boy, he
> worked for a shoe repairman named Dan MacKay. Dan
> was a devoted believer in Christ who desired to bring
> glory to God through his work. Young Harry's job was
> the monotonous task of pounding the water out of soaked
> pieces of cowhide for shoe soles. One of MacKay's unscru-
> pulous competitors down the street eliminated the process

---

1   James Strong, *Strong's Expanded Exhaustive Concordance of the Bible*, Gr. 1567.

of pounding the water out of the soles. This saved time during the shoemaking process, but it also meant the customer would have to come back sooner for a repair. Harry didn't understand why MacKay went to all the trouble of removing water out of the soles, but McKay's response was unwavering.

"Harry," he said, "I do not cobble shoes just for the [money] I get from my customers. I am doing this for the glory of God. I expect to see every shoe I have ever repaired in a big pile at the judgment seat of Christ, and I do not want the Lord to say to me on that day, 'Dan, this was a poor job, you did not do your best here.' I want Him to be able to say, 'Well done, good and faithful servant.'"[2]

And This Crown Ain't No Tooth

Perhaps it has never entered your mind that enduring temptations is something that God has promised to reward. It almost seems more fitting for God to reward great feats of faith, trust, and obedience. But that's exactly what enduring temptations entails. When you find yourself being drawn toward sin, your decision not to give in to it demonstrates the fact that you believe God's warning to turn away from it. Choosing to do what is right in place of what is wrong shows you trust that God knows best. And ultimately, by acting on your faith and trust, you demonstrate obedience.

It's reassuring to know that we do not need to infer that God rewards those who endure temptations through faith. In other words, we're not just somehow extrapolating this truth from the Hebrews 11:6 passage that we've been examining. While it would be a legitimate conclusion to draw from the text, Scripture actually teaches this reality explicitly: "Blessed is the man who endures temptation; for when he has been approved, he will receive the crown of life which the Lord has promised to those who love Him" (James 1:12). There it is. God's unwavering

---

2   Mark Hitchcock, *Heavenly Rewards: Living with Eternity in Sight* (Eugene, OR: Harvest House, 2019), 123–24.

and undeniable assurance that He rewards those who stand strong and endure in the face of temptations.

Have you ever wondered why so many men not only give in to sexual temptations but are also willing to sacrifice the most important things in life for such a short-lived pleasure? We discussed this in depth in the last chapter, but I'm always astounded at how so very common this is among men. But as a man, I also completely understand the intensity of sexual temptations. Is it any wonder then that God rewards endurance in this traumatizing arena?

It's important at this juncture that I clarify what James was referring to when he spoke of "the crown of life." We find this same crown mentioned in Revelation 2:10, when Jesus addressed believers in the ancient church of Smyrna, and also in the context of faithful endurance by those who were tested with times of intense tribulation. Bible scholars have noted that Scripture speaks of five different crowns: the imperishable crown (1 Corinthians 9:25), the crown of rejoicing (1 Thessalonians 2:19), the crown of righteousness (2 Timothy 4:8), the crown of glory (1 Peter 5:4), and the crown of life. The Greek word for "crown," *stephanos*, used in both James 1:12 and Revelation 2:10 can refer to a reward or to a laurel wreath. This crown may be tied to the bema seat of Christ from 2 Corinthians 5:9–10, which we discussed in an earlier chapter. Again, the bema seat is likened to a judge's seat in ancient athletic competitions from which competitors received their rewards.

In light of this, it's important to know that this crown of life is not the same as God awarding us salvation on the basis of our works. Scripture is clear that salvation is a free gift, that we are saved by grace through faith, and that this reward is most definitely not based on our own righteous deeds (Ephesians 2:8–9). So this crown of life is not salvation but indicates eternal rewards of sorts, which God grants to Christians who have demonstrated faithfulness as they fought their way through the battlefield of temptations in life.[3]

What exactly are these rewards? How will they enhance our eternal existence? What benefits do they provide? We obviously don't know the definite answers to these questions. However, we do know the dispenser

---

3   Jeremy Myers, "What Is the Crown of Life?" Redeeming God, May 30, 2018, https://redeeminggod.com.

CROWN

of such rewards, and that should be enough to send a jolt of euphoric excitement through the core of our being. The excitement should spring from our knowledge of God's character and perfection. Understanding that He is love, we know that these gifts will be exceedingly good. And more than that, knowing that He's perfect, we realize that He can only give perfect gifts.

Even though we don't know for certain what exactly our heavenly rewards will be, J. Dwight Pentecost gave a good description of what they might possibly entail:

> Inasmuch as reward is associated with brightness and shining in many passages of Scripture (Daniel 12:3; Matthew 13:43; 1 Corinthians 15:40–41, 49), it may be that the reward given to the believer is a capacity to manifest the glory of Christ throughout eternity. The greater the reward, the greater the bestowed capacity to bring glory to God…Capacities to radiate the glory will differ, but there will be no personal sense of lack in that each believer will be filled to the limit of his capacity.[4]

Spiritual Anti-itch Cream

When we explored how evangelism is an important aspect of walking in the Spirit in chapter 13, we focused on the tragedy of Christians forfeiting certain rewards by failing to maintain faithfulness in their conduct. However, the focus in this chapter has been on the joy of receiving eternal rewards as we choose the path of sacrifice by obeying God and turning away from the sexual sins that are displeasing in His sight and devastating to our soul. It's crucial that we remind ourselves of this when we're being vexed on every side and hounded by the devil, the flesh, and the world to scratch what sometimes feels like a chronic and unbearable itch.

While we may feel a twinge of guilt for looking forward to heavenly rewards and allowing them to be one of the incentives for resisting sexual temptations, I assure you that this guilt is completely irrational. We have nothing to feel guilty about when we get excited and motivated

4   J. Dwight Pentecost, *Things to Come: A Study in Biblical Eschatology* (Grand Rapids, MI: Zondervan, 1958), 226.

by the things that God Himself has promised are rewards for our obedience. Paul gave us a glimpse of this beautiful truth and included us in it when he spoke about his perseverance in the fight of faith and the completion of his race—tying it all together with the glorious reward that awaits him and us in God's kingdom: "I am already being poured out as a drink offering, and the time of my departure is at hand. I have fought the good fight, I have finished the race, I have kept the faith. Finally, there is laid up for me the crown of righteousness, which the Lord, the righteous Judge, will give to me on that Day, and not to me only but also to all who have loved His appearing" (2 Timothy 4:6–8).

What a beautiful way for Paul to describe the end of his life's journey in the faith. He likened himself to a drink offering being poured out. This symbolized the final act of the offering ritual under the Old Testament sacrificial system, when the priest would pour out a cup of wine right next to the altar after a sacrifice was made (Numbers 15:1–10; 28:4–7).

While Paul was indicating that the end was near for him, his positive description of the nature of his exit was the real focus. He didn't just fight, but he fought the good fight. He didn't just run his race, but he also finished it. He didn't just have faith, but he also kept it until the very end. And so, having conducted himself in this way and having crossed the finish line victorious in Christ, for Christ, and through Christ, Paul was undoubtedly looking forward to the exceedingly great reward that the Lord had reserved for him in His kingdom. And while this was Paul's delight at the end, it was no doubt one of the motivating factors throughout his pilgrimage as a believer—a pilgrimage that was unquestionably fraught with temptations at every turn.

He's No Cosmic Killjoy

It's important to remember that heavenly rewards are not the selfish by-products of man's creative imaginings. God is not a cosmic killjoy who is stingy with His children. He revels in giving us good gifts and is zealous to fill our lives with joy, both temporal and eternal. It would do us good to remember this powerful scriptural truth: "He who did not spare His own Son, but delivered Him up for us all, how shall He not with Him also freely give us all things?" (Romans 8:32).

In describing the source of heavenly rewards, Woodrow Kroll eloquently articulated their true origin: "Rewards are God's doing. They were his idea, not ours. God is the one who developed the rewards, determined the criteria for awarding them, and demonstrated his grace by providing them for faithful service. Rewards arise from the heart of God...Don't rob God of the joy of being a rewarding heavenly Father because you tell him you don't care. You should care. It's okay to think about your heavenly reward. God does."[5]

Indeed, the creator of our heavenly rewards does most certainly think about them, and He wants us to think about them as well. Moses is a great example of a man who walked in faith—not only believing that God is but also believing that God is a rewarder of those who diligently seek Him. Moses sought God well as he fled from sin and looked to the reward of the great rewarder: "By faith Moses, when he became of age, refused to be called the son of Pharaoh's daughter, choosing rather to suffer affliction with the people of God than to enjoy the passing pleasures of sin, esteeming the reproach of Christ greater riches than the treasures in Egypt; for he looked to the reward" (Hebrews 11:24–26).

So how, then, should all this play out in real life? What do you do when your hormones are intensely raging and you find yourself submerged in the sea of sexual temptations, getting hit by one monstrous wave after another every time you resurface for air? First, you realize that compared to eternity, this seemingly endless and vexing crucible is very short-lived. Then, you remind yourself that in contrast to this transient season, the freedom that awaits you is eternal. Finally, you will yourself into meditating on the truth that your choice to endure your temptations now will secure for you priceless, everlasting rewards that you will enjoy forever in that coming state of eternal freedom. You couple this with saying to yourself, *Crown: envision endurance ensuring eternal enrichment.*

Our journey started with creation, then moved on to cross, crisis, and crown. We will now venture into the exploration of crowd.

---

5   Woodrow Kroll, *Facing Your Final Job Review: The Judgment Seat of Christ, Salvation, and Eternal Rewards* (Wheaton, IL: Crossway, 2008), 44.

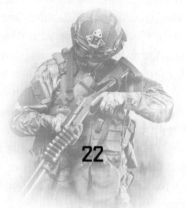

22

CROWD

DO AS THE DEPARTED DID
AND DON'T DISPENSE DEVASTATION

Running While Seated

Wait…what? Are my eyes deceiving me? A woman was autographing books by holding a pen between her teeth. That sight was new and unusual to me. Of course, I had heard of her and her condition, but seeing her in person and watching her in action was an altogether different matter. But it wasn't just what she was doing that mesmerized me. It was also her glowing countenance and the otherworldly joy that emanated from her despite the exceptionally challenging circumstances that she lives with.

Before she needed to use a wheelchair, like the one I saw her sitting in at the Christian Booksellers Association convention, Joni Eareckson Tada loved hiking, swimming, playing tennis, and horseback riding. She was a vivacious young woman with boundless energy and a heart that yearned for adventure. But on a tragic day in 1967, at only seventeen years of age, Joni dove into the Chesapeake Bay, miscalculating the shallowness of the water, and fractured her vertebrae. She emerged from that water a quadriplegic, permanently paralyzed from the shoulders down.

Now, imagine that this was you and try to grasp the devastation of that moment when you suddenly realized that your limbs no longer followed your brain's commands. That every physical activity you ever enjoyed was permanently stripped from you. That you could never again describe yourself with the word *independent*. No more running or walking or standing or writing or holding anything—ever. Even brushing your teeth on your own or feeding yourself or personally tending to your body's most basic needs would most likely require the assistance of someone else.

While Joni admittedly went through a very dark season of depression and hopelessness, as the Lord started working on her heart, something in her began to change. Her consciousness of eternity and its value slowly awakened. And with that awakening came the realization that even in her extraordinarily challenging state, God was good and worthy of praise, worship, and absolute surrender. Joni understood that the Lord had not forsaken her, that she had a purpose to fulfill, and that what seemed like a catastrophe presented a unique opportunity through which she could serve and glorify God by impacting others.

Only someone who has had a paradigm shift of epic proportions could face constant struggles and suffering and still say, "My weakness, that is, my quadriplegia, is my greatest asset because it forces me into the arms of Christ every single morning when I get up."[1]

Just when it seemed like Joni's circumstances couldn't get worse for her, this dear sister found herself in an intense battle with cancer. But look at what she said about it in an Instagram post a few years later: "When I received the unexpected news of cancer from my oncological surgeon, I relaxed and smiled, knowing that my sovereign God loves me dearly and holds me tightly in His hands. What good is it if we only trust the Lord when we understand His ways? That only guarantees a life filled with doubts."[2]

And what does a life lived like that, by someone battling such extreme suffering, do for us? Does it not inspire us and rouse us to greater feats of faith and trust and commitment to the Lord?

Years after first meeting Joni, we were privileged to have her as a guest on a program that I was cohosting for our ministry's YouTube

1   Eryn Sun, "Joni Eareckson Tada on Wilberforce Award, 'Better Off Dead than Disabled' Mentality," *Christian Post*, March 16, 2012, https://www.christianpost.com.

2   "Joni Eareckson Tada Receives New Cancer Diagnosis," Joni and Friends, November 19, 2018, https://joniandfriends.org.

channel. And there she was, still pressing on, still touching others, still glorifying the Lord, still shining brightly with a contagious love for Jesus, and still running her race—even in a wheelchair.

Follow the Crowd

As I consider Joni's powerful example, I'm reminded of a rousing exhortation that God divinely gave us in the book of Hebrews: "Since we are surrounded by so great a cloud of witnesses, let us lay aside every weight, and the sin which so easily ensnares us, and let us run with endurance the race that is set before us" (12:1).

Perhaps as you noticed that this is the opening verse of Hebrews 12, you thought to yourself, *What in the world is he talking about? Who is this "cloud of witnesses" that the author of Hebrews randomly brought up?* I sincerely appreciate the challenges faced by those who gifted the church with chapter and verse divisions in the Bible. I can't even begin to imagine what a monumental task it must have been to figure out the appropriate places to break things up. However, knowing that there were no chapter and verse breaks in the original biblical writings, we would need to back up into Hebrews 11 to understand who the cloud of witnesses is.

Hebrews 11 has been famously dubbed the Hall of Faith. In this chapter, we find the names and laudable deeds of those who dared to take God at His word and trust Him with their lives amid some of the most challenging circumstances imaginable. We find such greats as Abel, Enoch, Noah, Abraham, Isaac, Jacob, Sarah, Joseph, Moses, and Rahab. After highlighting the extraordinary things that God did in and through these godly saints of old, the author of Hebrews wrapped up the chapter with this inspirational, soul-stirring, and convicting declaration:

> What more shall I say? For the time would fail me to tell of Gideon and Barak and Samson and Jephthah, also of David and Samuel and the prophets: who through faith subdued kingdoms, worked righteousness, obtained promises, stopped the mouths of lions, quenched the violence of fire, escaped the edge of the sword, out of weakness were made strong, became valiant in battle, turned to flight the armies of the aliens. Women received their dead raised to life again.

Others were tortured, not accepting deliverance, that they might obtain a better resurrection. Still others had trial of mockings and scourgings, yes, and of chains and imprisonment. They were stoned, they were sawn in two, were tempted, were slain with the sword. They wandered about in sheepskins and goatskins, being destitute, afflicted, tormented—of whom the world was not worthy. They wandered in deserts and mountains, in dens and caves of the earth.

And all these, having obtained a good testimony through faith, did not receive the promise, God having provided something better for us, that they should not be made perfect apart from us. (11:32–40)

It is immediately after this—in the very first verse of the very next chapter—that we see those powerful words from Hebrews 12:1. This is that specific cloud (or crowd, as some have translated it) of witnesses. They are those who reveled in triumphant victories and who persevered amid great trials of suffering. But all of them—despite their particular set of circumstances—have "obtained a good testimony through faith" (11:39). The inspired text of Scripture is telling us that it is they who now surround us, God's people who are carrying on the faith today. It is their good testimony that should serve as the example of how we run the race that God has set before us.

I have no doubt that the great cloud of witnesses played a part in inspiring Joni to continue running her race, and she is now a living part of those same witnesses who continue to encourage us. This brings to mind the insightful truth conveyed in the opening chapter of 2 Corinthians: "Blessed be the God and Father of our Lord Jesus Christ, the Father of mercies and God of all comfort, who comforts us in all our tribulation, that we may be able to comfort those who are in any trouble, with the comfort with which we ourselves are comforted by God" (1:3–4).

Hebrews says that the fact that this great cloud of witnesses exists and lived such lives of vibrant faith while on earth is the very reason why we are to "lay aside every weight, and the sin which so easily ensnares us" (12:1). They demonstrated the ultimate in self-denial, self-control, and absolute surrender. They've shown us that, through faith, it's possible to be victorious conquerors and to preserve a good testimony while facing seemingly insurmountable circumstances and even temptations (as we're told in 11:37 that they "were tempted"). These witnesses "obtained a good testimony through faith" (v. 39), and because we serve the same God and are indwelt by the same Spirit, we can do it too.

A Weighty Matter

I find it interesting that the author of Hebrews referenced the weights and sins that ensnare us immediately after mentioning the cloud of witnesses. In fact, he told us that it's expressly *because* we are surrounded by the noteworthy examples of those who have gone before us that we should "lay aside every weight" (12:1). I wonder if, along with inferring that the exemplary finish to their race gives us hope that we, too, can complete our own course with excellence, the Hebrews author may also have been cautioning us not to mar their legacy with the stain of sin. This would rob future generations of believers from gaining another inspiring witness in that great, collective cloud and bring reproach on the gospel before the eyes of a watching world.

It's noteworthy that the text makes a distinction between two indisputably negative elements: weights and sin. While we would expect sin to be mentioned, why was it necessary for the author of Hebrews to highlight weights alongside sin, and what exactly are these weights? Because sin is more clearly discernible to us and no serious Christian would deny that sin is a stumbling block that we must cast off, we will focus our attention on the weights.

It's clear, at face value, that the weights are stifling elements, considering the fact that this Scripture passage calls us to cast them aside and to instead run our race with endurance. The race imagery that this passage uses helps us to imagine what the author means by the word *weights*.

When someone runs in a race, they have two primary objectives: to finish the race and to finish first. Of course, it's impossible to win without reaching the finish line, so the second objective is really the primary goal, and it presupposes the first. Paul exhorted believers to have the ambitious attitude of a winner when running their spiritual race: "Do you not know that those who run in a race all run, but one receives the prize? Run in such a way that you may obtain it" (1 Corinthians 9:24).

Of course, we must understand the real thrust of this within its proper context. Our aim is not to compete with other believers as though the faith were some sort of contest where we try to outdo one another. The focus is really the composure and mindset with which we are to run our race. We should have the same drive to finish well that a competing runner has. We should go all out, hold nothing back, and let nothing slow us down. We should run like someone who very seriously wants to win.

With all this in mind, it makes total sense that we would want to get rid of anything in our lives that would in any way slow us down. While I already talked about the foolishness of abiding by minimalistic standards in a previous chapter, I think it's important to revisit that topic here.

If your heart is genuinely set on honoring the Lord by running the race He's called you to run—with an aspiring winner's attitude—then you wouldn't be asking yourself how you could run while at the same time wearing your beloved cozy sweater, your most comfortable pair of jeans, and your favorite Doc Martens boots. And let's not forget your huge I-never-leave-home-without-it coffee mug and your five-gallon, dual-insulated, vacuum-sealed water bottle. Is it forbidden for a marathon runner to wear and carry those things during a race? Of course not. But what kind of impression does this give the spectators, and what outcome will it produce?

Those watching you run by will immediately recognize that you're not very serious about the marathon, nor are you committed to it. As far as the result of the race goes, it would be an absolute miracle if you even made it one mile through the race encumbered by all these items. And if somehow you did reach the finish line, it may be right around the time they're starting the marathon again the following year.

When it comes to what you can participate in while running your race of sexual purity, a number of things may be permissible for you—things that aren't necessarily sins. You might watch particular movies, TV programs, and online videos. Perhaps you can listen to certain songs and talk show programs. Maybe you can engage in a few affectionate activities with your girlfriend or fiancée. But you ultimately have to ask yourself if these things help you to run your race with greater endurance. Or are some of them weights that encumber you and slow your pace?

You may very well conclude that some of the elements listed do legitimately benefit you as you negotiate your course, but are you willing to cast off the ones that don't? Are you determined to say the following? *I've seen the great cloud of witnesses who have gone before me walk in victory and triumph. I've seen the harrowing trials, unimaginable sufferings, and intense temptations they endured through faith. I serve the same God, I'm filled with the same Spirit, and, by His grace and strength and help, I can and will do the same.*

A Life-Changing Lesson from a Lovely, Little Lady

I now want to turn our attention toward a different crowd. Not the one that went ahead of us and left us an inspiring example to follow but rather the one that stands in front of us—the crowd that sometimes looks to us as their examples, who often follow in our footsteps, or who are, at the very least, influenced by our lives to some degree. I distinctly felt the weight of this reality after an intense experience with my daughter many years ago.

It would be hard to ever describe a shout as normal, but this one was especially distinct and disturbing—even more so because it came from my wife at a late hour. It jarred me out of a deep sleep around 4 a.m. and sent me running wildly down the hallway toward our seven-year-old daughter's bedroom. I stumbled into the room half-awake to find my bride in a state of utter and desperate panic. And when I looked at our precious firstborn child, I immediately understood why. Julia's eyes were rolled back in her head, her body was shaking violently, and she was foaming from her mouth.

My wife and I became a tumultuous whirlwind of activity as we frantically tried to revive our daughter and figure out what was going on. When our attempts proved unsuccessful, we quickly called 911. The paramedics arrived in a few moments, and they informed us that our girl was experiencing a seizure.

The hours that followed that traumatic incident are a blur. We were praising God that our daughter was alive, but we were also shocked and frazzled, and a barrage of questions swirled in our heads. *Is Julia okay? What triggered this? Are seizures going to be a lifetime battle for her? Is she going to have to take heavy medications? Did she suffer brain damage?*

And every question seemed to beget a hundred more questions. While it's hard to remember everything that unfolded between the arrival of the paramedics and the emergency room doctor finally giving us his findings, there is one thing that I will never forget for the rest of my life.

Following the flurry of activity, I was sitting at the side of Julia's hospital bed while she lay there unconscious. Her tiny body was hooked up to multiple tubes as machines monitored her vitals and gave her necessary fluids and medications. Her body looked almost lifeless to me. As I sat there in the hush of that surreal moment with tears streaming down my face, I was overwhelmed by the thought that we could have lost our little girl.

Amid my emotional exhaustion, I remember clearly thinking that if she needed my eyes to see, I would immediately rip them out and give them to her. If she needed my heart, I would gladly tear it from my chest for her sake. If she needed my blood to stay alive, I would drain every drop from my body to preserve her life. Nothing would stop me from sacrificing myself to save my precious daughter. There was no question whatsoever about that.

As I fixated on those things, another thought rose to the surface of my mind and completely redirected my focus. I remember asking myself this question: E.Z., *you're willing to die in order to preserve Julia's life, but are you willing to die to yourself in order to further godliness in her?*

That was a very poignant and sobering wake-up call. However, this wasn't a "come to Jesus" moment for me. Not only was I already saved at the time, but I was also a pastor who was joyfully serving the Lord and walking closely with Him. Instead this question was a challenge for me to carefully watch my life and conduct and to remember that the decisions I made in the face of future temptations had the potential to impact my precious daughter—and for that matter, everyone within my sphere of influence.

Watching You Like a Hawk

We must consider the massive crowd of people that God has providentially placed in our lives, a crowd made up of a wife, children, parents, siblings, nieces, nephews, aunts, uncles, cousins, neighbors, employers, employees, coworkers, mentors, mentees, friends—and I'm sure a lot of other associations that I haven't even thought of. It is highly likely that among these groups are both believers and unbelievers. And while the degrees of closeness between you and all the people in your life will vary, the overwhelming majority of people that you interact with will know that you profess to be a follower of Christ. It's this very fact that should make us take inventory of the tone and tenor of our lives and remember that our actions have massive ripple effects. As believers, we are representatives of Christ, and everything we do reflects on our Lord and the gospel that we claim has transformed our lives. There is nothing that wounds the souls of others more than hypocrisy. Now this doesn't mean that every time a Christian sins, he is being a hypocrite (though it can be true in some instances), but nonetheless, many will perceive it as that. One of the most common and heartbreaking complaints about Christians is that they are hypocrites.

I remember sharing the gospel with a young man outside of a coffee shop many years ago. After I wrapped up my message to him, he looked at me with a very pained look on his face and said, "All my life growing up, my dad was a pastor, and never once did I hear him talk about God outside of church." His statement nearly knocked the wind out of me. Even as I recall that encounter today, it's hard not to get emotional about it. What this dear soul was saying, in so many words, is that there was a huge disconnect in his dad's life between what he professed in one place and how he lived in another—and it really hurt him.

Now, can you imagine the devastation and confusion experienced by those who know someone who speaks a lot about God all the time yet is living in secret sexual sin the whole time? What do you think this would do to a young teenager who is convinced that his dad is an honorable man? What about the wife who has devoted her whole life to a husband whom she thought was upholding the vows that he made to her as they stood at the altar? What about those who trusted that their leader was a man of integrity and uprightness? And what of the lost souls who discover that the person who passionately proclaims the gospel to them is not living a life that conforms to its life-changing truths?

Dealing a Life-Giving Death Blow

Can you say with our sister Joni Eareckson Tada that your weaknesses drive you into the arms of Jesus every morning? Are you stirred by her tenacious persistence and that of others like her who dared to press on amid challenging circumstances with the primary goal of inspiring others? Do you remember the example of the great cloud of dearly departed in the revered Hall of Faith of Hebrews 11, those who demonstrated to us how to triumph victoriously through faith and how, by that same faith, to persevere amid great temptations and trials of suffering? Are you moved in the core of your conscience when you consider the prodigious influence that you wield over the men, women, and children who surround you?

If you answered those questions in the affirmative, then you must take immediate action—the type of action that will result in you laying aside every weight and sin that ensnares you and running your race with endurance. This will then lead you to evaluate the way you think, the places you go, the things you watch and listen to and participate in. You will have to decide whether you're willing to overhaul your life and deal a death blow to the egocentricity that causes you to satisfy the interests and well-being of no one but yourself.

As you take this proactive and decisive action, it will help to train your mind by regularly ruminating on the biblical truths that we highlighted in this chapter. You must always remember the crowd that's made up of the cloud of great witnesses who went before us and left us a stellar example to follow. And you can never forget the crowd of precious souls all around us—the ones we should seek to guard against devastation by living in sexual purity and the ones for whom we should, in turn, leave a stellar example to follow. And while doing that, you can repeat this abbreviated exhortation to yourself: *Crowd: do as the departed did and don't dispense devastation.*

After soaking our hearts and minds in creation, we headed toward the glorious cross. We then endured a disheartening yet sobering gaze at crisis and were encouraged when we considered the hope found in the truths of crown. Having just immersed ourselves in the eye-opening realities of crowd, we will now head toward the last C, which is both our final and most important stop—Christ.

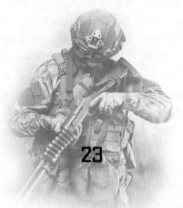

23

CHRIST

SEEK THE SWEET SAVIOR FOR STRENGTH, SATISFACTION, AND SYMPATHETIC SUPPORT

I Didn't Even Know My Own Name

I had no idea that our family friend's casual visit to my childhood home would forever change a major aspect of my life. After all, his visits were frequent, and while our time with him was always enjoyable, it never led to anything revolutionary. But little did I know how different this particular visit would be. While we were sitting around in our living room pleasantly chatting, Simon, who was in his late twenties at the time, casually looked over at little ten-year-old me and said, "You know that your name is easy, right?"

Huh? Not really, I thought. Tom, Bob, Joe, and Tim are easy names—but Emeal? I don't think so. It's important to note that I used to spell my name E-m-i-l-e back then, and many would horribly mispronounce it—"Emily" being my least favorite mispronunciation of all.

"What do you mean?" I asked.

"Yeah," he replied. "Your name is easy. Emeal—E and Zwayne—Z. They are your initials: E.Z."

I can't even begin to describe the euphoric bliss that invaded my heart at that moment in time. You have to keep in mind that this was 1985. It was smack dab in the middle of the breakdancing revolution that took the world by storm. This was the era when every cool kid had a catchy nickname like Gizmo, Turbo, and Uzi. I was sure it had to be Christmas, the Fourth of July, and a royal coronation all at the same time. I felt like I was given a hundred trillion dollars during a massive fireworks show while simultaneously being crowned king of the world.

I remember immediately running out of the house and rapturously declaring to my friends, "My name is E.Z.! My name is E.Z.! Start calling me E.Z." Well, that didn't work. They couldn't quite kick the Emile habit. But when I went to summer school shortly after that and pretty much no one on that new campus knew me, it was game on! At the start of the first day of class, the teacher said, "When I call your name, let me know if you happen to go by a nickname." Glory! I became the most popular kid on campus. But after summer school, it was back to Emile. However, my family moved to a different area when I was twelve, and no one at my new school knew me, so I was back to the cool life—and it's been E.Z. ever since.

I know what you're thinking, and that's exactly why I wrote everything you just read. Let me trip you out by magically revealing the thought that just went through your mind: *How in the world could you have been ten years old and never realized that your initials were E.Z.?*

Um…

And that's all I've got.

My wife, Rachel, and I must share the same befuddling deficit. The night before I wrote this, she sent a group text to our family and said, "I just realized that I have the word *ache* in the middle of my name. Literally just right now. How does a person go their whole life and not notice something like that?"

Now that's definitely something to ache over. My shameless boast is that I made my discovery a few decades before she made hers. Give me a trophy!

I'm not sure when my father-in-law, Ray Comfort, made the earth-shattering discovery about his name, but at least his revelation was a spiritual one. He loves telling people that he is always in prayer—twenty-four hours a day, 365 days a year. And he's right. *Ray* is always in p*ray*er.

These absurd stories about how oblivious my wife and I were regarding certain aspects of our own names are meant to illustrate that we can be extremely close to something and still not realize significant things about it. Think of the countless times we said, wrote, read, heard, and thought about our own names, yet the obvious completely eluded us—for a very, very long time.

Look Here, Mister

Growing up in a Catholic home, I heard the name of Jesus Sunday after Sunday. I saw that crucifix hanging in our church more times than I could count. I said Christ's name every night for years, and I rattled it off during my memorized prayers. And I called myself by that same name as I regularly referred to myself as a Christian. But it's frightening to consider how very little I knew about the person of the Savior and how so ignorant I was about the significance of the cross.

When God finally saved me on that divine August evening in 1991, the blinders fell from my eyes, and I was blown away by how much I had missed about my precious Savior. I was in awe over all that He had done to redeem my wretched and undeserving soul. This was the ultimate paradigm shift. It was one single revolutionary moment that undid years of deception, waywardness, and spiritual blindness.

Our default tendency is to run as far away as possible from Jesus whenever we find ourselves struggling with sexual sin, especially if we've fallen into it. Our sense of guilt and shame deceives us into thinking that the Lord wants nothing to do with us. If this is the perception that you have of Christ, then you've definitely missed some extremely important truths about His nature, His character, and His heart toward you as His child. And you've also overlooked some extremely important aspects of His glorious gospel.

One of the most crucial and indispensable things that you must understand about achieving victory over sexual sin is that you must do it through the strength and support of your Savior. You can never forget that apart from Him, you can do nothing (John 15:5). Jesus must be your everything. Glorifying Him must be your ultimate motive for walking in purity. Bringing His heart pleasure and being a vessel of honor in His hand must be the fuel that propels you forward on the highway of holiness.

In the previous chapter, we examined Hebrews 12:1 and homed in on our calling to remember the great cloud of witnesses that surrounds us while at the same time laying aside the weights and sins that ensnare us. I want us to now turn our attention toward the very next verse that instructs us on how to run our race with endurance: "Looking unto Jesus, the author and finisher of our faith, who for the joy that was set before Him endured the cross, despising the shame, and has sat down at the right hand of the throne of God" (Hebrews 12:2).

"Looking unto Jesus." Something about those words deeply touches me. They're indicative of hope and help and rescue. They're a reminder that the one who said He would never leave me nor forsake me (Hebrews 13:5) and who would be with me always, even unto the end of the age (Matthew 28:20), has remained faithful to His promise. It means that He who knit me together in my mother's womb (Psalm 139:13), who knows the number of hairs on my head (Luke 12:7), and who understands my darkened heart far better than I ever could (John 2:24–25) still loves me despite my utter wretchedness (Romans 5:8). It's a loud and clear declaration that He knows my frame and remembers that I am dust (Psalm 103:14), yet He still will never reject me or abandon me (Psalm 48:14).

Recalling those glorious truths intensely increases my desire to look unto Jesus. And nothing makes me want to flee sin more than when my gaze is steadfastly fixed on Him. This is all buttressed by the reminder that Jesus Himself is the "author and finisher of our faith." What comfort, consolation, and reassurance! He Himself initiated our faith, and being that He always finishes what He starts, we can rest assured that He will graciously see to it that what He started in us He will fully complete. Because as "author," He is literally the "founder" and "originator" of our faith, the one who inaugurated it and established it.[1] And if He authored, founded, and originated our faith, then it naturally follows that He will also be its "finisher," or its "completer," "consummator,"[2] and "perfector."[3]

---

1 *Mounce's Complete Expository Dictionary*, "Archēgos," StudyLight.org, accessed September 7, 2023, https://www.studylight.org.

2 James Strong, *Strong's Expanded Exhaustive Concordance of the Bible*, Gr. 5051.

3 *Thayer's Expanded Greek Definition*, "Teleiōtēs," StudyLight.org, accessed September 7, 2023, https://www.studylight.org.

The Sinner's First Aid

With the theme of looking unto Jesus firmly fixed in our minds, we'll back up a number of chapters in the book of Hebrews and reinforce the truth that we've been contemplating. I honestly don't know where I would be as a Christian if I were not intimately familiar with this life-altering passage: "We do not have a High Priest who cannot sympathize with our weaknesses, but was in all points tempted as we are, yet without sin. Let us therefore come boldly to the throne of grace, that we may obtain mercy and find grace to help in time of need" (Hebrews 4:15–16).

Unlike the earthly high priests under the old covenant, who made sacrifices to God for the sins of His people, our eternal High Priest, Jesus, was Himself the willing sacrifice for our propitiation. But dissimilar to the earthly sacrifices that had no connection to the people until they were sacrificed on their behalf and that ceased to exist once they were sacrificed, Jesus, in our place, lived the perfect life that we couldn't live and rose again from the dead after He was crucified for us. And yet, as He lived that perfect life by flawlessly keeping the law of God during His progressive journey toward the cross, He faced a massive number of temptations. While never sinning, of course, He experienced every form of temptation that is common to mankind.

But perhaps you're thinking, *How would it have been possible for Jesus to be tempted to watch pornographic videos online when that technology didn't even exist in His time?* While it's true that watching online pornography would not have been a temptation for Jesus, the foundational temptation that is related to that activity is lust. And sure enough, Jesus would have certainly been tempted to lust. Moreover, we can name many similar examples in this regard. But how amazing it is to think that because Jesus experienced temptations, His heart toward us as we wrestle with the temptations that assail us is not one of frustration or exasperation or anger but one of sympathy.

Fathom that! Christ feels for you in your time of weakness and struggle. In other words, He has pity, understanding, and patience toward you. And then, in direct opposition to your inclination to run from Him and hide in shame over your constant battle with sin, He calls you to come to His throne of grace and to do so not with fear and hesitation but boldly. He says that it's at that throne where He will dispense mercy and grace to help you in your time of need.

Hebrews 2 gives us a deeper insight into this glorious truth: "In all things He had to be made like His brethren, that He might be a merciful and faithful High Priest in things pertaining to God, to make propitiation for the sins of the people. For in that He Himself has suffered, being tempted, He is able to aid those who are tempted" (vv. 17–18). What a revolutionary and soul-comforting truth. God willingly became like us not only to redeem us but also to specifically come to our aid during our moments of temptation—in faithfulness and with mercy.

Jesus never kicks His people when they're down. He doesn't ghost them, dissociate from them, or give up on them. In fact, in one of his descriptions of Christ, Matthew referenced an Old Testament prophecy about the Messiah from Isaiah 42:1–4, which highlights a very touching description of how He relates to sinners: "A bruised reed He will not break, and smoking flax He will not quench, till He sends forth justice to victory; and in His name Gentiles will trust" (Matthew 12:20–21).

Instead of tossing out a bruised reed as useless, the Savior mends it and restores its firmness and sturdiness. Instead of snuffing out a smoldering wick that's barely kept alive by a slowly fading ember, He gently blows on it until He reignites its burning flame.

One Must Walk Worthy of the Most Worthy One

The realization of Jesus' gentleness, patience, and tender care toward us amid our struggles should not only stir us to draw closer to such an unspeakably merciful, gracious, and loving redeemer, but it should also rouse us to determine to live in a way that honors Him. We've already discussed the importance of walking in a manner that is worthy of the gospel and all that this entails; however, Scripture also calls us to another worthy walk: "Walk worthy of the Lord, fully pleasing Him, being fruitful in every good work and increasing in the knowledge of God" (Colossians 1:10). This means that we need to live in such a way that our conduct aligns with the worthiness of Christ, the one whom we call Lord.

Think of the crippling grief that the apostle John must have felt when, during the mind-blowing revelation that God gave him, he "wept much" (Revelation 5:4) because no one in heaven or on earth was found worthy to open the scroll with its seven seals. But then consider the rapturous joy that must have invaded his being when the elder said to him, "Do not weep. Behold, the Lion of the tribe of Judah, the Root of David, has prevailed to open the scroll and to loose its seven seals" (v. 5). Could there have been a more fitting scene than the one that followed that glorious declaration?

> When He had taken the scroll, the four living creatures
> and the twenty-four elders fell down before the Lamb, each
> having a harp, and golden bowls full of incense, which are
> the prayers of the saints. And they sang a new song, saying:
>> "You are worthy to take the scroll,
>> and to open its seals;
>> for You were slain,
>> and have redeemed us to God by Your blood
>> out of every tribe and tongue and people and nation,
>> and have made us kings and priests to our God;
>> and we shall reign on the earth." (vv. 8–10)

A realization of Christ's worthiness always leads to an appreciation of what He did to redeem us, the infinitely undeserving. It unveils layer after layer of the unfathomable depths of His boundless and multidimensional love. He didn't shed the blood of bulls or goats or rams to redeem us to God, but He willingly shed His own blood. He did this not for His worthy children or friends but for His unworthy and reprehensible enemies, rebels who spurned, maligned, and blasphemed His holy name.

Fear-Filled, Faithful Followers

Peter appropriately linked our understanding of the value of Christ's blood with how we determine to live out our lives as pilgrims on this earth: "If you call on the Father, who without partiality judges according to each one's work, conduct yourselves throughout the time of your stay here in fear; knowing that you were not redeemed with corruptible things, like silver or gold, from your aimless conduct received by tradition from your fathers, but with the precious blood of Christ, as of a lamb without blemish and without spot" (1 Peter 1:17–19).

When Christ redeemed us, He rescued us from one of the most destructive elements of our godless lives—aimless conduct. Aimlessness is indicative of a purposeless and directionless existence. It conjures up imagery of a lost wanderer going around in circles with no destination in view. He lives in an endless cycle of monotonous wastefulness. Having been delivered from this misery by the most precious substance that has ever existed—the holy blood of Christ—we should loathe even the slightest thought of ever returning to aimless conduct.

In light of what He did for us, how could our hearts not burn with the kind of unquenchable love for Him that should make us want to run as far away as possible from even the slightest hint of sexual immorality? This is the natural outcome of the holy fear that Peter referenced—a fear that is steeped in awe, respect, reverence, and honor and that teaches us to depart from evil (Proverbs 16:6).

As we do this, Jesus becomes more and more precious to us. Our heart's capacity to love and appreciate Him expands. We joyously identify with these beautiful sentiments that Spurgeon penned about our precious Jesus:

> I bear witness that never servant had such a master as
> I have; never brother such a kinsman as he has been to
> me; never spouse such a husband as Christ has been to
> my soul; never sinner a better Saviour; never mourner a
> better comforter than Christ hath been to my spirit. I want
> none beside him. In life he is my life, and in death he shall
> be the death of death; in poverty Christ is my riches; in
> sickness he makes my bed; in darkness he is my star, and in
> brightness he is my sun; he is the manna of the camp in the
> wilderness, and he shall be the new corn of the host when
> they come to Canaan. Jesus is to me all grace and no wrath,
> all truth and no falsehood: and of truth and grace he is *full*,
> infinitely full.[4]

---

4   Charles H. Spurgeon, "May 10, Evening," in *Morning and Evening*, accessed August 30, 2023, https://www.biblegateway.com.

He's Got the Mightiest Touch

When I was a newer Christian, my heart leaped for joy when I read this verse in Peter's first epistle: "Whom having not seen you love. Though now you do not see Him, yet believing, you rejoice with joy inexpressible and full of glory" (1 Peter 1:8).

As the legendary apostle spoke about the sentiments of God's people toward Jesus in this way, all I could do was exclaim, "Amen!" from the very core of my being. This is exactly how I feel about the lover of my soul. Though I have not yet seen Jesus with my naked eye, there is no one in all existence whom I love more than Him. And despite the fact that I still can't see Him now, my heart is constantly rejoicing over Him with inexpressible and glory-filled joy.

There's no greater earthly example of this kind of love than in the life of Helen Keller. Helen, born in 1880, became blind, deaf, and mute at the age of two. She was trapped in an isolated world of darkness. Due to her inability to communicate or normally interact with others, her frustration incrementally intensified until it reached a boiling point. As the years of her childhood passed, she became more and more erratic and incorrigible. Her heartbroken parents did everything they could to get her the help she needed. They hired one expert after another to find a solution for her situation. Her case was so extreme and her behavior so outrageous that everyone eventually gave up, urging her parents to send Helen to an institution. But one day, a very determined and unrelenting woman entered Helen's life. Her name was Anne Sullivan.

Unlike others who came before her, Anne was unwilling to surrender in her battle for Helen's rescue. As she persisted in teaching Helen the building blocks of communication in the face of what seemed like insurmountable odds, the day finally came when her unwavering determination paid off. After many unsuccessful attempts, Anne finally devised a brilliant teaching method of sign language that surprisingly unlocked the world of communication for Helen. This massive breakthrough radically revolutionized Helen's life, and she was forever changed. She went on to become a university graduate, an author, a lecturer, and although I don't agree with everything she supported, there's no denying she is one of the most celebrated and inspirational figures who has ever lived.

As you can imagine, Helen Keller and Anne Sullivan formed a deep and insoluble bond. In fact, they became practically inseparable. Wherever Helen went, there was her faithful teacher, interpreter, confidante, and best friend. Anne resolutely remained by Helen's side until the day that Anne died, October 20, 1936.

What amazes me most about this epic account is that Helen Keller never once saw Anne Sullivan's face and she never once heard her voice. She primarily experienced her through one distinct sense—both literally and figuratively—the sense of touch. Helen was so deeply touched by Anne's love, care, and sacrificial service that, even though she never saw her face or heard her voice, she loved no one on earth more than Anne, and she undoubtedly rejoiced over her with joy inexpressible and full of glory.

With that illustration fresh in our minds, let's read Peter's powerful words again: "Whom having not seen you love. Though now you do not see Him, yet believing, you rejoice with joy inexpressible and full of glory" (1 Peter 1:8).

Perhaps now you can understand why it is that I can't help but shout, "Amen!" to those divine words. It's because Jesus has touched me unlike any other. When everyone else had given up on me, considered me hopeless, helpless, and irredeemable, He swooped down with undeterred and unwavering love and rescued me from myself and from the hot and holy wrath of God that I so justly deserved. How could I not be forever enraptured with a Savior as inexplicably magnificent as Him?

The famed church father Augustine of Hippo was able to beautifully articulate what the true Christian feels in his heart about Christ— the second person of the triune Godhead, God the Son. Having lived a godless life that was steeped in the excesses of debauchery, sexual promiscuity, and vain worldly pursuits, Augustine was one day utterly conquered by the saving grace of God and radically transformed into a new creation. Being that Augustine was forgiven much, he most certainly loved much, and Jesus became everything to him. My inner man is overcome every time I read these captivating words that Augustine penned about his love for God:

But what do I love when I love my God? Not the sweet
melody of harmony and song; not the fragrance of flowers,
perfumes, and spices; not manna or honey; not limbs such
as the body delights to embrace. It is not these that I love
when I love my God. And yet, when I love Him, it is true
that I love a light of a certain kind, a voice, a perfume, a
food, an embrace; but they are of the kind that I love in
my inner self, when my soul is bathed in light that is not
bound by space; when it listens to sound that never dies
away; when it breathes fragrance that is not borne away on
the wind; when it tastes food that is never consumed by the
eating; when it clings to an embrace from which it is not
severed by fulfillment of desire. This is what I love when I
love my God.[5]

Only someone who has experienced the new birth can relate to a
description like that, which so profoundly captures what it's like to love
Christ, whom Augustine called, "My Lord and my God," like Thomas the
Apostle (John 20:28). And as true and poetic as those rousing words are,
they still fall short of fully conveying what it's like to be in close union
with the one who is life itself.

Think of His impact on hearts and minds and lives and souls and
the entire course of human history when Jesus graced this planet with
His divine presence. The historian Philip Schaff captured this well:

Jesus of Nazareth, without money and arms, conquered
more millions than Alexander, Caesar, Mohammed, and
Napoleon; without science and learning, he shed more
light on things human and divine than all philosophers
and scholars combined; without the eloquence of school,
he spoke such words of life as were never spoken before or
since, and produced effects which lie beyond the reach of
orator or poet; without writing a single line, he set more
pens in motion, and furnished themes for more sermons,
orations, discussions, learned volumes, works of art, and

5   Augustine of Hippo, *Confessions*, trans. R. S. Pine-Coffin (London: Penguin Books, 1961), Book X.6.

songs of praise, than the whole army of great men of ancient and modern times.[6]

Not So Yum Yum for My Tum Tum

When we fully grasp who Christ is and all that He is meant to be to the believer, it really helps us understand why Christians sometimes stray into sexual immorality. Jesus made this astounding claim about Himself in the gospel of John: "I am the bread of life. He who comes to Me shall never hunger, and he who believes in Me shall never thirst" (6:35). Our Lord is speaking here of spiritual sustenance. He is declaring Himself to be the ultimate provision for all mankind's spiritual cravings. When someone is regenerated and becomes joined to Christ, the spiritual appetite that God has placed in every human being is satisfied by the spiritual sustenance that He has designed that appetite to be satisfied with. And that sustenance is the very person of Jesus. However, in the same way that people enter the process of starvation when they cease to eat physical food, so it is that we enter the process of spiritual starvation when we cease to feast on spiritual food—on the Bread of Life—Christ Himself.

If you live in the Western world, starvation probably is the furthest thing from your mind. You likely don't wake up in the morning gripped by fear over whether you'll be able to find enough to eat for the day. If anything, because of the overabundance of food that's available to them, many people in advanced nations are preoccupied with trying to discipline themselves to eat less because of the negative impact that their constant overeating has on their bodies. But the United Nations reports that 489 million adults around the world are undernourished and 122 million children suffer from hunger.[7] All throughout the annals of human history, famines have claimed millions of lives. And in many cases, those who find themselves in the dire straits of famine end up eating things you can't even imagine. In actual accounts of starvation, people are reported to have eaten things like grass, leaves, tree bark, insects, rodents, and domesticated pets.

6   Dr. Philip Schaff, *The Person of Christ: The Perfection of His Humanity Viewed as a Proof of His Divinity* (New York: Charles Scribner, 1866), 21, https://www.ccel.org.
7   "World Hunger Statistics," The Barbecue Lab, last updated September 2023, https://thebarbecuelab.com.

In one of the most harrowing stories of starvation, author Piers Paul Read wrote about a Uruguayan rugby team, along with their friends and family, whose plane crashed in the Andes in October of 1972. Out of the forty-five passengers, only sixteen survived the crash. After exhausting the food they scrounged up from around the plane's strewn wreckage, the survivors ended up eating the dead bodies of their friends and loved ones in order to preserve their lives.[8]

Who in their right mind would ever eat such things—grass, leaves, tree bark, insects, rodents, pets, and other human beings? The answer is that no one in their right mind would eat such things under normal circumstances. However, those who enter the process of starvation find themselves under the influence of an altered state of mind as they transition through four different stages.

It all begins with *deprivation*. Whether voluntarily or involuntarily, a starving person is deprived of the normal, healthy sustenance that provides their body with the nutrients that it needs. But we can handle being deprived of proper food for only so long before we enter the next harmful stage—*desperation*.

It's here that things take a major shift in a dangerous direction. As hunger acutely intensifies, reason fades to the background, and a hyper-anxious urgency to find satisfaction takes over. Detestable things that we would otherwise never have considered for consumption suddenly look appetizing.

Desperation incrementally builds until it is uncontrollable, and *deviation* becomes inevitable. This is where we start to depart from a normal, healthy diet and begin to consume the unimaginable. Substitution becomes the norm, and little by little, our taste buds' preferences are altered. What once was appetizing to us fades from our memory, and the detestable perversely becomes a delight.

Once deprivation, desperation, and deviation have all fully run their course, we end up in the final and tragic stage of *deterioration*. After consuming unhealthy and harmful elements for a prolonged period of time, our bodies succumb to their toxic effects. Breakdown is unavoidable as we start to physically deteriorate more and more with each passing day. Our body's systems shut down, and our organs begin to fail.

---

8   Piers Paul Read, *Alive: The Story of the Andes Survivors* (Philadelphia: Lippincott, 1974).

The Spiritual Sustenance That Satisfies

Spiritual starvation very closely mirrors physical starvation. Again, God has given all His people a spiritual appetite that is meant to be satisfied by Christ. We crave specific things in the spiritual realm, and Jesus is the only person who can properly satiate each and every one of those cravings—and He delights to do so. But when deprivation becomes our chosen course of action, desperation kicks in, and before we know it, we find ourselves on the slippery slope of deviation, quickly descending into the destructive abyss of deterioration. Unfortunately, we can expect no other outcome.

Perhaps you've never considered the fact that God has given you a spiritual appetite for a first-love relationship, for friendship, for treasure, and for pleasure. We might expect all these things to align solely with physical desires. But God's Word makes it clear that there is a spiritual dynamic to all these important elements and that we should, therefore, pursue spiritual satisfaction in Christ for them all. This is when the pursuit of fulfillment finds its most virtuous expression and where we truly live out God's optimal design and intention for our lives.

When speaking to the church of Ephesus in the book of Revelation, Jesus began by praising them for some of their virtuous deeds and attributes. But then He quickly confronted them with a very weighty and serious rebuke. Here are the Savior's piercing words: "Nevertheless I have this against you, that you have left your first love" (Revelation 2:4).

Of course, Jesus was speaking of Himself here. While space doesn't allow us to explore the details related to His exhortation, let's note the significant fact that God designed us to have a "first love" relationship with the redeemer of our souls. This perfectly coincides with Paul likening a husband's relationship with his wife to Christ's relationship with the church (Ephesians 5:31–32).

One of the most touching and heartwarming passages of Scripture in the gospel of John reveals something extraordinarily tender about the heart of Jesus toward those for whom He laid His life down. If you're a Christian, you would be hard-pressed not to be deeply moved by these eye-opening words: "Greater love has no one than this, than to lay down one's life for his friends. You are My friends if you do whatever I command you. No longer do I call you servants, for a servant does not know what his master is doing; but I have called you friends, for all things that I heard from My Father I have made known to you" (15:13–15).

Our Lord didn't just say that self-sacrifice is the greatest expression of love toward one's friends, but He also went on to demonstrate it by laying His life down for us. And then He made it clear that those to whom He has revealed truth from the Father are the ones that He actually calls friends. That longing for real and meaningful friendship that sometimes wells up inside you is not random or coincidental. The God who sent His Son to die for you, save you, reveal His divine truths to you through His glorious Word, and make you His friend is the one who intentionally birthed this desire in you. And once you've tasted that incomparable spiritual friendship with Christ, your soul will always deeply desire to experience it.

When we consider the one who had "nowhere to lay His head" (Matthew 8:20), who called some to "forsake all" in order to be His disciples (Luke 14:33), and who exhorted others to "sell what [they had]" and to follow Him (Matthew 19:21)—the last thing we could imagine is that He would then call people to accumulate treasure. But that's exactly what He did: "Do not lay up for yourselves treasures on earth, where moth and rust destroy and where thieves break in and steal; but lay up for yourselves treasures in heaven, where neither moth nor rust destroys and where thieves do not break in and steal. For where your treasure is, there your heart will be also" (Matthew 6:19–21).

Christ's ambition was never to discourage the pursuit of riches; rather, it was to encourage the pursuit of the right kind of riches. In fact, His desire is for His children to be ultrarich, abounding with the sort of wealth that would make Elon Musk look like the poorest homeless beggar who ever lived. But it's spiritual wealth that He has in mind for those whom He loves. It's the kind of wealth that matters, that is eternal, and that we can acquire only from His gracious hand.

And how exactly do we acquire it? Only by living lives of service for the sake of Christ, in the name of Christ, and for the kingdom of Christ. And we do this while being eternally minded as we seek the things above (Colossians 3:1–3). So you were made to be ambitious to possess things. As counterintuitive as this is to us, when we seek to have the right things while doing the right things, we'll long to do more of the right things and hunger to have more of the right things.

While we might find it difficult to overcome our preconceived notions that it's not natural to find satisfaction in Christ in the areas of a first-love relationship, friendship, and treasure, we probably consider it nearly impossible to accept the fact that we can actually find satisfaction in Him in the area of pleasure. Maybe this is because our fallen minds are so accustomed to associating pleasure with things that are sinful and taboo.

However, in John 15, after Jesus described Himself as the Vine and said that we, as His people, should abide in Him like branches, He concluded by saying that we should abide in His love through obedience in the same way that He abides in the Father's love. Here Christ highlighted once again His unity and oneness with the Father. But then He revealed why He unveiled these glorious truths to His disciples: "These things I have spoken to you, that My joy may remain in you, and that your joy may be full" (John 15:11).

I think it is safe to say that, for the Christian, joy is the very pinnacle of pleasure. And this pleasure is interrelated with abiding in Christ, which also unites us with the Father. This abiding in obedience naturally happens when we enter into and dwell in the Lord's presence. How else could abiding really happen?

Psalm 16 reinforces what is available for God's people in the ineffable beauty of His glorious presence: "You will show me the path of life; in Your presence is fullness of joy; at Your right hand are pleasures forevermore" (v. 11).

How then do we practically enter into the presence of Christ? We do it by seeking after Him as we passionately pursue Him through close communion and intimate fellowship. It finds its ultimate expression when we regularly sequester ourselves in holy seclusion and pour our hearts out before Him in heartfelt prayer—adoring Him, praising Him, thanking Him, and worshiping Him. This then begins to spill over into every arena of life, unlocking the realization of His holy presence in all places and at all times. And then we couple this with connecting with His heart through His eternal Word by joyously reading it, memorizing it, meditating on it, and crying out to Him to help us understand it and live it out.

When we function in the sacred and solemn awareness of His presence and experience the incomparable joy and pleasure that come from consistently abiding there, we realize that there is no other place on earth where we would rather be. We start yearning for it and the joyous pleasure it brings, like a fish that washes up on land longs for ocean water and like a bird in a cage longs for heavenly air.

A first-love relationship, friendship, treasure, and pleasure—these are all spiritual cravings that are a part of our God-given spiritual appetites, which only Christ can satisfy. But when we deprive ourselves of Christ Himself in any of these areas, we become desperate as the cravings intensify and overwhelm us. It's at this juncture that we find ourselves deviating as we substitute feasting on Christ with feasting on the physical filth of the world. Some of these things are not necessarily filth in and of themselves, but they can become that when they replace Christ and we turn them into idols in our lives.

When it comes to a first-love relationship, we find ourselves unnaturally looking for satisfaction in the wrong type of woman—perhaps an unbeliever or someone other than our wife or we turn the wife that we do have into an idol.

In terms of friendship, we turn to friendship with the world, associating and becoming partakers with those who hate God and who are diametrically opposed to everything that He stands for. Or we become possessive, insecure, and jealous within our Christian friendships.

In relation to treasure, we become consumed with the love of money, coveting everything in sight and hoarding every materialistic possession that we can get our hands on. And the more things we own, the more those very things own and dominate us.

In connection to pleasure, we seek to indulge in as many endorphin-releasing, adrenaline-inducing, and orgasm-producing activities as possible, especially as they relate to our sexual appetites. It's here where many men become ensnared by lust, pornography, and masturbation and give in to fornication and adultery. And while all these activities might at some point have seemed unthinkable to many men, this is where a starving soul turns. The words of the old proverb ring true: "A satisfied soul loathes the honeycomb, but to a hungry soul every bitter thing is sweet" (Proverbs 27:7).

Once we deprive ourselves of feasting on Jesus as our ultimate source of spiritual satisfaction, we become desperate. After we become desperate, we deviate and substitute the spiritual with the physical in these areas and many more. And the result inevitably is spiritual deterioration.

It's for this reason that we must never stop feasting on Christ as our greatest satisfaction. He must remain our most precious first love, our soul's closest and dearest friend, our life's most prized treasure, and the greatest pleasure that our heart could ever enjoy.

He's Got You Covered

I'm sure it's no secret to you by now that one of the main objectives in this book is to help men flee the sin of sexual immorality in all its various forms. And someone else long ago also wrote with the aim of keeping God's people from sinning. I'll let you read those words for yourself: "My little children, these things I write to you, so that you may not sin" (1 John 2:1).

Every genuine believer who has experienced the new birth unquestionably cares about the welfare of other believers. And if they don't, there's good reason to suspect that they were never genuinely born again. The apostle John, the one who was so close to Jesus that he laid his head on the Lord's bosom during the Last Supper, was no doubt overflowing with the love of Christ, which he personally experienced, when he wrote his divinely inspired epistle in order to direct God's children away from sin. He made it clear that the purpose for which he wrote to them was so that they would not sin. John stood at the foot of the cross and looked up at Jesus, who hung upon it and bore the sins of wretched sinners. John understood sin's ravages, and he saw firsthand the incalculable price that God chose to pay because of it. And so, he yearned for God's people to utterly forsake sin.

But what happens when men do yield to the lure of the devil, the flesh, and the world and give in to the sexual temptations that assault them? Is it curtains for them? Are they rejected, discarded, and left without hope? When we look at the second part of the verse, we see that John understood that it's inevitable that God's children would sin. After saying that he wrote to keep believers from sin, he immediately added,

"If anyone sins, we have an Advocate with the Father, Jesus Christ the righteous" (v. 1).

John wanted Christians to know that God has already established recourse to deal with any sins that we might ever commit. His explicit plea is this: *Don't sin.* However, his immediate counsel states, *But if you do sin, don't become undone. You're not cast down or cast out. You're not left without help or hope or forgiveness.* And why is this life-altering and soul-restoring reality possible? Because Jesus is our Advocate! The word for "advocate" in the Greek, *parakleton*, refers to a person who pleads someone else's case directly on their behalf. It carries the idea of one individual helping another. In fact, it's the same word that John uses four times in chapters 14, 15, and 16 of his gospel in reference to the Holy Spirit. And in each instance, *Paraclete* is translated as "Helper" in the New King James Version.

So John wanted us to know that Jesus is our helper when we sin. He's there to plead with the Father on our behalf, pointing to the wounds in His hands, feet, and side as a declaration that He has satisfied God's justice and paid for our sins with His own precious blood.

This means that Jesus' help for us extends beyond the Hebrews 4 realm of temptation that we already explored. He stands ready, willing, and desirous to help us when we give in to temptations and stumble into the realm of sin. When Paul wrote in his letter to the Ephesians about the abundance of spiritual riches that the believer has in the Savior, he made sure to remind us that we possess this priceless gem as a part of our inheritance in Christ: "In Him we have redemption through His blood, the forgiveness of sins, according to the riches of His grace" (Ephesians 1:7). It's on the basis of this glorious and foundational truth that John was able to say this to believers who stumble into sin: "If we confess our sins, He is faithful and just to forgive us our sins and to cleanse us from all unrighteousness" (1 John 1:9).

I find it interesting that John used the word *righteous* to describe our beloved Advocate (2:1). And this makes perfect sense when we consider what the Bible says about Jesus in multiple places:

- "Indeed I also count all things loss for the excellence of the knowledge of Christ Jesus my Lord, for whom I have suffered the loss of all things, and count them

as rubbish, that I may gain Christ and be found in
Him, not having my own righteousness, which is from
the law, but that which is through faith in Christ, the
righteousness which is from God by faith" (Philippians
3:8–9).

- "Of Him you are in Christ Jesus, who became for us
  wisdom from God—and righteousness and sanctification and redemption" (1 Corinthians 1:30).

- "He made Him who knew no sin to be sin for us, that
  we might become the righteousness of God in Him"
  (2 Corinthians 5:21).

He can forgive us of our sins and cleanse us from all unrighteousness because He is our Advocate. He's Jesus Christ the righteous, who has
become our righteousness and has made us the righteousness of God in
Him. He is indeed the propitiation (or satisfaction) for our sins (1 John 2:2).

Paul gave a more detailed description of what this propitiation
looks like when he wrote to the saints in Colossae: "You, being dead in
your trespasses and the uncircumcision of your flesh, He has made alive
together with Him, having forgiven you all trespasses, having wiped out
the handwriting of requirements that was against us, which was contrary
to us. And He has taken it out of the way, having nailed it to the cross"
(Colossians 2:13–14).

This means that our debt has been fully paid, our sins have been
completely forgiven, and the warrant for our arrest and eternal condemnation has been rendered null and void. As Paul so beautifully put it,
God has nailed our sin to the cross. It died with Christ. When He uttered
the words, "It is finished," He signaled our liberation from bondage and
ushered in freedom from the dominion and destructive power of sin in
the life of every redeemed and adopted child of God.

Few things hinder the Christian's growth more than wallowing
in self-condemnation. There's a radically misleading element attached
to it that deceives the believer into thinking that this behavior is
almost virtuous. But there's nothing virtuous about living out an irrational existence. And acknowledging that this sort of condemnation
is self-condemnation is exceedingly appropriate because it's certainly

not coming from God. That's what makes it irrational. God's redeemed children are inflicting themselves with something that doesn't even exist. Because as God's Word clearly declares, "There is therefore now no condemnation to those who are in Christ Jesus, who do not walk according to the flesh, but according to the Spirit" (Romans 8:1).

And just in case your condemning mind leads you to think that there is condemnation for you because there are times when you stumble into the flesh and fail to walk in the Spirit, Paul went on to clarify exactly what he meant: "You are not in the flesh but in the Spirit, if indeed the Spirit of God dwells in you" (Romans 8:9). The impetus of Paul's glorious announcement is that if you are indwelt by God's Spirit—meaning if you are born of God and are regenerate—you are in Christ, and there is no condemnation for you whatsoever.

So as much as you should seek never to sin, as much as you should hate sin and resist it and flee from it, when you do stumble into it, run to Jesus. Run to Him without hesitation. Run to Him boldly, urgently, and with complete abandon. He will never turn you away. He is your Advocate, your propitiation, your righteousness. He shed His precious blood for all the sins you would ever commit before you even existed to commit them. He demonstrated His love toward you in that while you were yet a sinner, Christ died for you (Romans 5:8). He has obliterated every article of condemnation against you and snuffed out the burning flames of hell that awaited you.

And if, after running to Him, you sin again, then run to Him again and again and again. No matter how many times you have sinned in the past or think you will sin in the future, every time you sin, run to Him—and never stop running to Him. Remember this: "In Him [you] have redemption through His blood, the forgiveness of sins, according to the riches of His grace" (Ephesians 1:7).

From A to Z

There is nothing more important in all life than for the child of God to fully grasp who Jesus really is. Understanding His nature, His attributes, His character, His ways, and His heart toward His redeemed people is paramount for any man of God who seeks to stand firm and fight victoriously in his battle against the devil, the flesh, and the world.

One of my favorite descriptions of Jesus is found in the book of Revelation. And what's most endearing to me about it is that this is how our Lord described Himself: "I am the Alpha and the Omega, the Beginning and the End, the First and the Last" (Revelation 22:13).

Jesus used the first and the last letters of the Greek alphabet to highlight something of utmost importance regarding who He is: He's the first and the last, the beginning and the end. This speaks of His fullness, His wholeness, His all-sufficiency.

Years ago, I came across this anonymous poem of sorts that greatly stirred my heart in the way it describes Jesus using every letter in the alphabet:

> To the artist, He is the altogether lovely One.
> To the builder, He is the chief cornerstone.
> To the chef, He is the Bread of Life.
> To the doctor, He is the Great Physician.
> To the educator, He is the master teacher.
> To the florist, He is the rose of Sharon and lily of the valley.
> To the geologist, He is the Rock of ages.
> To the horticulturist, He is the true Vine.
> To the intellectual, He is the wisdom of God.
> To the jeweler, He is the head of the church: the pearl of
>   great price.
> To the king, He is the Prince of Peace.
> To the lawyer, He is the judge of all the earth.
> To the manufacturer, He is the creator of all things.
> To the newsperson, He is the glad tidings of great joy.
> To the oculist (in search of the light), He is the Light of the
>   World.
> To the philanthropist, He is the gift of God.
> To the queen, He is the King of kings.
> To the rabbi, He is the Messiah.
> To the scholar, He is the truth.
> To the theologian, He is the author and the finisher of their
>   faith.
> To the undertaker, He is the resurrection and the life.

To the visionary, He is the revelation of God.

To the waiter, He is the one who came not to be served but to serve.

To the X-ray technician, He is the Word of God before whom all things are naked and bare.

To the youth, He is the life.

To the zealot, He is the Son of God for whom life is worth living.

While the writings of man are both flawed and limited and knowing that Jesus is infinitely more than all the inerrant and infallible biblical descriptions that the poem portrays Him to be, it's still a good reminder to us that, as He said of Himself, He is indeed the great "I AM" (John 8:58). As the God of the universe, He is the ultimate satisfaction for every spiritual desire He's given you. So feast on Him incessantly and look unto Him as you run your race with endurance, for He is indeed the author and finisher of your faith.

Make it your daily routine to unlock all the biblical truths in this chapter by saying to yourself, *Christ: seek the sweet Savior for strength, satisfaction, and sympathetic support.*

This completes our journey through the six Cs. From creation to cross, to crisis, to crown, to crowd, to Christ, we explored crucial elements of our battle plan against the schemes of our relentless enemies in our fight for sexual purity. We have one final weapon to examine—one that I'm sure you'll find extremely helpful and that will serve you well in your quest for victory.

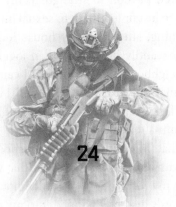

24

NOPE

Enough Already!

How are you doing in your struggle with pornography?" I asked the young man whom I was counseling. Unlike most of the guys I have counseled, this one had not gone off the deep end into the dark and destructive world of porn, but he was definitely tempted to do so. He assured me that he had been standing strong in this area. I went on to follow that question with another question. "How are you doing with lusting after women that you see when you're out and about every day?"

"Not well," he confessed—with a tinge of defeat in his voice. As I began to both encourage and exhort him in this regard, I sensed a deep zeal for purity well up inside me. The reality of how often so many of us men are bound and dominated by sexual lust overwhelmed my heart with an urgency to see this radically change.

I looked at this dear soul sitting in front of me and said, "Sometimes we just need to say to ourselves, *This is enough! I'm done with this!* And then we need to make a commitment not to give in to lust by uttering the word *nope* out loud."

This seemed to resonate with my young friend, and it definitely stirred something in my own heart. I walked away from that counseling session with a renewed passion to strengthen my defenses against the insidious temptation to lust or to give in to sexual immorality of any kind.

The next morning, after I left my house to head to my office, I saw a couple of very scantily dressed women jogging near my car as I drove through my neighborhood. As soon as I caught sight of them in my periphery, I automatically exclaimed, "Nope!" I instantly felt a strong resolve rise up in my heart, and it flooded my whole being with a mixture of unwavering determination and satisfying joy.

I remember that as soon as this happened, I wished I could somehow come up with a meaningful acrostic that would help focus my mind and strengthen my resolve anytime I'm tempted to lust. About five seconds later, four words instantly popped into my mind:

Not
One
Peek
Even

I wish someone could have snapped a picture of my face at that very second. I felt like I had struck gold, and the beaming smile on my face made that very evident. Beyond the fact that I theoretically believed that I had acquired a tool I was confident would help other men and me, my joy resulted from the immediate benefit that I experienced in real time. I'm at a loss for words to describe it, but that special moment was both distinct and sublime. It bordered on the euphoric in the spiritual realm.

Stop "Peeking" Your Interest

Peeking is where it all starts. And peeking will definitely result in piquing your interest when it comes to the area of lust. Whether we do it with our physical eyes or with our mind's eye, a peek—even a quick one—most often leads to a stare. In many cases, we do not have the opportunity to stare at a woman whom we quickly peeked at. Whether we passed one by, saw an image of one on a billboard or in a quick advertisement, conjured up an old memory of one, or fabricated one out of thin air in our mind, taking that intentional, second peek at a woman—again, with our physical eyes or with our mind's eye—can lead to that leering stare in our thoughts and imagination. And a stare, of course, will inevitably lead to the sin of lust.

Now as we consider the sin of lust, Jesus' sobering words on the subject should rouse us to run as far away as possible from indulging in even the slightest peek: "You have heard that it was said to those of old, 'You shall not commit adultery.' But I say to you that whoever looks at a woman to lust for her has already committed adultery with her in his heart" (Matthew 5:27–28).

If there's anything we should know well about ourselves as fallen men, it's the fact that we have an affinity for constantly trying to justify the unjustifiable. It goes something like this:

- *I know that it's not best to go to a Las Vegas show that's full of exotic dancers, but I'm trying to reach my cousin with the gospel, and he really wants me to go with him.*

- *I realize that this commercial has a very immodest woman in it who's wearing tight leggings and moving around seductively, but the exercise machine she's advertising looks very interesting. I need to see if it's something I may want to purchase.*

- *I can immediately tell from the thumbnail that this YouTube video has a woman in it that I'm going to struggle with lusting over, but it will be good for me to watch it anyway because that will help me build up my resistance.*

- *Yeah, it's evident from my peripheral vision that the lady walking in my direction is barely wearing any-thing, but I think I might know her, so I should probably take a good look at her—just to make sure.*

- *It has been many years since my ex-girlfriend and I broke up; I'm sure I can safely reminisce about some of the innocent times we had together without my mind venturing into the sinful times.*

Let me be blunt with you here, my friend: don't play the fool by deceiving yourself into thinking that you can take this naive approach and escape without scars. You know you can't because you've tried and never succeeded (at least not consistently), and you'll never succeed at it now or in the future.

Each day of your life will be riddled with countless lust traps wherever you go. How you train your mind, your heart, and your eyes will be the deciding factor between constant ensnarement and liberating freedom. We are resolute and stubborn creatures of habit, and as the old saying goes, "You'll always be who you've always been if you always do what you've always done." Something drastic in your default functioning has to change. This is where I firmly believe the NOPE principle will be a valuable asset to you.

It's not a difficult task to find stubborn men roaming the planet. They're more abundant than light bulbs in Las Vegas, golf balls in Palm Springs, and palm trees in Florida. But the sad and unfortunate thing is that most of them are stubborn in the wrong direction and about all the wrong things. Pastor and writer Scott Hubbard shed light on what men should really be stubborn about, what they need to be saying no to, and how they should be saying it:

> The "No" of self-control is not the calm "No" of a wedding
> RSVP. It is the terrible "No" of self-denial—of refusing
> to gratify the inner beast that barks for satisfaction. Self-
> control can feel like severing an arm or tearing out an eye
> (Matthew 5:29–30).
>
> But God's word doesn't merely describe the anguish
> of self-control. God meets us in that dreadful moment,
> and tells us how we can meet our sin at the door, hear its
> desperate pleas, and still say "No."[1]

Time to Get Sassy

If you think about it, you'll realize that there is an edgy flare associated with the word *nope*. It comes loaded with tenacity and attitude. There is a big difference between responding to someone's request with a bland no (akin to the mild type of no mentioned in Hubbard's quote) and doing so with a sassy nope. The former gets the job done without much fanfare,

---

1   Scott Hubbard, "You Can Say No to Sin," Desiring God, August 28, 2018, https://www.desiringgod.org.

but the latter blows a trumpet, detonates a nuclear bomb, and—for good measure—drops a resolute exclamation mark the size of Mount Everest on the landscape of your resistance.

No other attitude will do when dealing with the temptation to lust. A flavorless no is insufficient. Our will must bellow out a thunderous nope. When possible, I recommend saying the word aloud. If you're in a setting where it's possible only to whisper it, then do that. If even a whisper is not possible, then mouth the word. I think physically expressing the word with our mouth increases our level of commitment and creates a greater sense of self-accountability that reinforces and drives our determination.

If you discover that the employment of NOPE in a given situation is not helping you much, use it while simultaneously meditating on the six Cs. This powerful combination can help to radically reinforce your resistance. I also encourage you to go the extra mile and forge your own custom weapons that will further help you in your battle. Each man's life circumstances differ from others', and so I'm sure with some focused thought and prayer, you can formulate something that will be specifically applicable and extremely beneficial to you.

For example, as a married man with kids and grandkids, when I say NOPE in times of temptation, I combine it with five declarations associated with love and directly correlated to five fingers on one of my hands. As a citizen of God's kingdom, I imagine myself extending my hand toward a plow, as Jesus referenced in Luke 9:62, and determining not to look back toward any sexual temptation that would lure me away from my God. As I envision myself reaching out to grab the plow, I say the following five things, in successive order, as I systematically wrap each of my corresponding fingers, one by one, around the handle: "Not One Peek Even—because I love my *Lord*, I love my *lady* (my wife), I love my *lineage* (my children and grandchildren), I love His *lambs* (other Christians), and I love the *lost* (unbelievers). And then I hold on tightly with a firm and unyielding grip.

If you're really serious about fighting like a man, brother, then you're going to have to be exceedingly firm in your determination. You'll also need to be brutal about how you deal with what comes across your eyes and what crops up in your mind. I have found very few words that have stirred my soul in this regard more than these:

> Every thought in your mind needs to be filtered.
>
> If you are going to survive this war, you need to be a domineering, controlling, micro-managing tyrant when it comes to your thought life. Any and all thoughts outside of God's Word, you take captive, shut up, and expel. You give those thoughts no time. No mental real estate. No free pass. You throw those thoughts into prison. No, better yet, you send them straight to solitary confinement. And when you're done, you throw away the keys.[2]

A Lesson to Learn From— Not a Loony, Legalistic Law

Now it's important to note that this NOPE thing is not some sort of law that you're obligated to uphold. There's no biblical mandate that tells you to say a crafted mantra aloud—or in any other fashion—in order to have victory over sexual temptations. You may think that using the NOPE method of resistance is just strange and not for you. I can completely understand that and would encourage you to throw my suggestion out the window if that's how you feel about it. I've had to do that with a number of recommendations that people have given to me over the course of my life.

It's best to see the NOPE method as a tested, practical tool that may aid you in breaking the habit of chronic lust. I've been both amazed and delighted by how many of the men with whom I've shared NOPE have told me that it has revolutionized this area of their life.

If we were to draw on somewhat of a biblical example of this sort of thing—though, of course, it's by no means a perfect or binding parallel—it would be the principle of meditation that I already touched on. Again, among other things, meditation involves muttering truth to oneself. We can see King David doing this sort of thing in one of the most treasured psalms: "Why are you cast down, O my soul? And why are you

2   John Mark Comer, *My Name Is Hope: Anxiety, Depression, and Life after Melancholy* (Portland, OR: Graphe Publishing, 2011), 133.

disquieted within me? Hope in God; for I shall yet praise Him, the help of my countenance and my God" (Psalm 42:11).

If you desire to adopt this practice in your life but are unsure about saying NOPE aloud, you can at least try saying it in your head. Regardless of what angle you take when using the acrostic, if you consistently employ it, you'll find that it will automatically echo in the corridors of your mind and influence you to do what's right in moments of temptation.

Even Cooler Than a Cucumber

The last thing this tool should do is make you anxious and paranoid just because you see a woman or encounter a sexual temptation, erratically shifting your eyes and frantically shaking your head as you run around everywhere screaming, "Nope!" The wise man will not allow himself to become undone in the face of temptation. He won't panic and repeatedly tell himself to stop thinking of a pink elephant because he knows that this will only make him think of one all the more. No, instead, he'll turn his gaze toward God, implement his predetermined battle plan, calmly but firmly say no to sin, confess any sinful desires in his heart, and go on his way rejoicing in the Lord.

Listen, there's absolutely nothing wrong with looking at a pretty woman and appreciating her beauty. How else would any man be able to pursue a relationship with a woman and get married? But we all know ourselves, and we recognize the difference between innocent appreciation—even admiration—and sinful lust. We can all detect when our senses are heightened and we're more susceptible to veering off into dangerous territory. It's at those times that it's crucial for us to strengthen our resolve and guard ourselves from dishonoring the Lord.

The bottom line is that the less lust-inducing imagery you give your mind and flesh to feed on, the better. It really comes down to wisdom, sobriety, and self-control. Calmness is also a key factor. Realize that there is no limit to what can enter your fallen mind and what it's capable of conjuring up. Remember your three relentless enemies—the devil, the flesh, and the world—are constantly bombarding you with all sorts of temptations in the form of thoughts and images. You're not at fault for these elements that assail you, but you are responsible for the sinful desires in your heart.

You have a choice as to whether you will give in to lust when you encounter these things. As Martin Luther said, "You cannot prevent the birds from flying in the air over your head, but you can prevent them from building a nest in your hair."[3] So knowing this should keep you extremely calm and composed. You don't have to act erratically, feel anxious, and condemn yourself when temptations dangle in front of you. It's no more your fault than it is a fish's fault when a baited hook drops in front of it. But just like the fish, there's no one to blame but yourself if you take the bait.

Do the Job Like Job

I've always found Job's example of sexual integrity to be both convicting and inspiring. When God Himself says about an individual that "there is none like him on the earth," that he's "a blameless and upright man," and that "he fears God and shuns evil" (Job 1:8), we would do well to take notice. Here is what this exemplary giant said about his determination to avoid lusting in his heart: "I have made a covenant with my eyes; why then should I look upon a young woman?" (Job 31:1).

Ponder that for a moment. Job didn't just casually say, "I'll try not to lust." He was so serious about it that he described it as a covenant. A covenant is a formal, sacred, and irrevocable promise. After making that solemn declaration, Job then asked a piercing question, "Why then should I look at a young woman?" It's almost as if though Job was saying, *Hey, if I'm so serious about sexual purity that I've taken the drastic step of covenanting with my eyes, why in the world would I be casual with what my eyes look at and, in turn, do the very thing that would violate my covenant?*

May we not only be convicted and inspired by Job's example of sexual fidelity, but may we also determine to passionately follow it. What would prevent us from covenanting with our own eyes not to look lustfully at women? If we followed the wise exhortation in the book of Proverbs, we would deliver ourselves from the destructive ravages of sin

---

3   Martin Luther, *Luther's Catechetical Writings: God's Call to Repentance, Faith, and Prayer*, trans. John Nicholas Lenker, vol. 1 (Minneapolis, MN: Luther Press, 1907), 305.

and spare our souls from accumulating the lasting scars that waywardness leaves behind:

> Let your eyes look straight ahead,
> and your eyelids look right before you.
> Ponder the path of your feet,
> and let all your ways be established.
> Do not turn to the right or the left;
> remove your foot from evil. (4:25–27)

And if you find yourself in the crosshairs of a seductive woman who is proactively seeking to lure you into her web of immorality, may you take heed to this sobering imperative from God's precious Word: "Do not lust after her beauty in your heart, nor let her allure you with her eyelids" (6:25).

Say Nope and You Will Cope with Hope

Remember that lust begins with a first impure peek—whether it's a physical or a mental one. So when you're handling your daily affairs and attractive women cross your path, direct your lips and your heart to exuberantly declare, "NOPE!" When you're driving down the street and encounter a billboard plastered with smut, "NOPE!" When you're flicking through the television channels and come across something salacious, "NOPE!" When you're surfing the web or interacting with social media and inappropriate pictures pop up, "NOPE!" When you pass by an adult bookstore or you come across a pornographic magazine or your mind is invaded by sexually obscene images, "NOPE! NOPE! NOPE! Not now. Not ever. Not One Peek Even!"

CONCLUSION

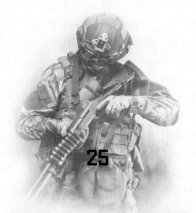

25

RUN THAT BY ME
ONE MORE TIME

A Friendly Reminder

Well, there you have it—a bold, biblical battle plan for personal purity. My question to you now is will you confidently step up and vigorously fight like a man?

Think about how many lectures you've heard in school, how many conversations you've had with people, how many sermons you've listened to, articles you've perused, and books you've read over the course of your lifetime. Now ask yourself how much of that information you can still remember. Chances are, probably not very much of it. My prayer is that this book will not be another one whose message you will quickly forget.

As I'm sure you've detected after reading the preceding pages, I'm extremely passionate about the pursuit of sexual purity. I'm heartbroken by how sexual immorality has ravaged men, destroyed families, and marred the testimony of the gospel. And I long to effectively serve men by giving them a solid tool that will help them experience victory over this insidious sin.

While it's unlikely that you and I have ever met, our journey together through this book connects us in a very special way. I took the time to write it, and you took the time to read it. Both of us now share in the same stream of knowledge. I know a lot about how your heart and mind work when it comes to sexual struggles because I share in your manhood and your sinful nature. You know quite a bit about my life because I unveiled a lot of it to you across the many pages through which you have doggedly traveled. We've been through a lot together, and in a way, we've sort of become friends. This bond that we've forged makes me eager for you to have a lifetime of benefit from whatever truths in this book align with God's Word. It would pain me deeply to think that after investing several hours of your time—perhaps over the course of days, weeks, or months—there's a possibility that you could forget most of what you've learned.

In light of that, I thought it would be most effective to use this last chapter to briefly recap the salient points we've covered. While I tried my best to make the contents of this book memorable, it's still hard for the mind to capture that much information without some sort of refresher. While I think that rereading the book in its entirety would go a long way in helping you to more effectively retain the truth it contains, I've also chosen to highlight and summarize its key points here. That way you can refer to this chapter repeatedly and, in a short amount of time, reengage with the most helpful portions of the book's message.

Preventative Preparedness

Real men heed the call to fight tenaciously for what matters. They conduct themselves honorably and uprightly, denying themselves and doing difficult things for the sake of love. They guard and protect those whom they genuinely care for, and they're willing to lay down their life in the process. Men are constantly engaged in a war for sexual purity. Failing to recognize this fact leads to dire consequences.

Life is not a resort; it's a battlefield. You don't travel through this world on a luxury cruise ship into an atmosphere of leisure but on a battleship into a realm of combat. Your greatest form of protection against your fiendish foes is the strategy of preventative preparedness. This "peace through strength" posture will help minimize offensive assaults against you and free you up to serve the Lord while maintaining a cautiously defensive disposition.

Your Three Main Enemies

Your three main enemies in your battle for sexual purity are the devil, the flesh, and the world. Each of them has a specific offensive against you. You must understand their schemes and counter them with your own battle plan for victory.

The Devil

Being mindful that Satan is the Father of Lies is essential. You must always guard yourself against the three main weapons that he will employ against you—the same ones he used at the dawn of creation against Adam and Eve—discontent, disbelief, and deification.

Discontent: You must battle discontent with gratitude and thanksgiving, raising up your shield of faith to quench Satan's lies and avoiding covetousness (which is idolatry) at all costs. Remembering the overwhelming blessings with which God has showered you will enable you to shake the groundless suspicion that the Lord is withholding something good from you. This will empower you to trust that He knows best, cause you to rest in His goodness, and help you to find contentment in the gifts He's lavished you with, both in time and for all eternity.

Disbelief: When the Enemy hits you with disbelief about the serious consequences of sexual sin, you must hit back with your knowledge of the unchanging character of God. You have to stand firm on the foundation of His immutable truth and on the guarantee that you will always reap what you sow (Galatians 6:7–8). You acknowledge the fact that Scripture distinctly singles out sexual immorality as an egregious sin with grave consequences, you dare to examine yourself to see if you are genuinely a Christian (2 Corinthians 13:5; 2 Peter 1:10), and you determine that on the day of judgment, you do not want to be an "I wish I would have" person but an "I'm glad I did" man.

Deification: While attempting to drop his nuclear bomb of deification on you, Satan will lure you to try to usurp God's throne by seeking autonomy and by determining for yourself what is right and wrong in the arena of sexual pleasure. You must heavily arm yourself with the understanding that the most foolish and dangerous thing you could ever do is to seek to rule over your own life—considering that some people can't even stop their own hiccups. You must remember the fate of all who sought to deify themselves and ascend the throne of God—those like Satan, Adam and Eve, Nebuchadnezzar, and King Herod Agrippa I. You choose instead to bow your knee in submission to the sovereign and loving Lord of the universe, realizing that His ways are always perfect and always best for you.

The Flesh

The flesh is our second enemy that will seek to dominate us as it entices us with every unlawful sexual pleasure that appeals to our carnal nature. And our carnal nature is exactly what the flesh is—that part of our being that was corrupted at the fall in Eden. It's that inherited corruption that is diametrically opposed to everything that is holy, righteous, and pleasing in the sight of God. Galatians tells us that the flesh and the Spirit are constantly at war with one another and that the way to have victory over the flesh is to "walk in the Spirit" (Galatians 5:16–17).

When God's Word speaks of someone "walking in the spirit," it's referring to being a person who is controlled by the Spirit of God. One of the ways that you can most effectively be controlled by God's Spirit is by involving yourself in the things that God's Spirit is involved in. When we look at Scripture, we discover that there are four main areas that God's Spirit is distinctly at work in: prayer, God's Word, fellowship, and evangelism. As you joyfully immerse yourself in these wonderful Spirit-saturated privileges with which God has gifted you, you will consequently starve your flesh and its carnal desires. This will allow you to experience victory over the power of the flesh and its destructive influence.

All this comes down to how your mind is geared and where your mind is set. Romans 12:2 commands us not to be "conformed to this world" but to be "transformed by the renewing of [our] mind." Colossians 3:1–2 instructs us to "seek those things which are above, where Christ is" and to "set [our] mind on things above, not on things on the earth." This will determine whether you are controlled by God in the various areas of your life or by people, thoughts, emotions, and circumstances.

Those who are controlled by people, thoughts, emotions, and circumstances are like a television that has multiple remote controls with codes that correlate to the code in the television's receptor device. As these different elements press various buttons, specific signals are sent out that solicit the person to respond in accordance with the fruit of the flesh. When our minds are set on earthly things, we will immediately respond to those signals.

The man who seeks the things that are above and sets his mind on them is like a TV that has only one master remote control with a code that correlates to the code in its receptor device. As people, thoughts, emotions, and circumstances push their buttons and send out signals that solicit responses that are in keeping with the fruit of the flesh, the eternally minded person is not affected by those signals. But when God simultaneously presses the buttons on His master remote, sending out signals that solicit from His child responses that are in keeping with the fruit of the Spirit, the eternally minded and Spirit-controlled man yields in obedience to God's holy will.

Here are the questions you need to sincerely ponder: Will you succumb to the enticements of your carnal nature and yield to its sexually charged signals—thereby bearing the flesh-saturated fruit of adultery, fornication, uncleanness, and lewdness? Or will you surrender to the control of the Holy Spirit and yield to God's righteous signals, thereby bearing the Spirit-saturated fruit of patience, goodness, faithfulness, and self-control?

The World

Our third and often most underestimated enemy is the world. When I speak of the world in this context, I'm not talking about the planet that we live on but rather the fallen and corrupt system of man that is in rebellion against God, His reign as the sovereign ruler of the universe, and His transcendent, immutable, moral law. It's this very world that God's Word tells us not to love: "Do not love the world or the things in the world. If anyone loves the world, the love of the Father is not in him" (1 John 2:15). It's also the one that we're exhorted to never befriend: "Adulterers and adulteresses! Do you not know that friendship with the world is enmity with God? Whoever therefore wants to be a friend of the world makes himself an enemy of God" (James 4:4).

As we make it our aim to run as far as we can from loving the world and befriending it, we must first be keenly on our guard against the world's "wisdom." Mantras are often the medium through which the world delivers its foolish counsel. Three of these most popular and sinister mantras are "Follow your heart," "God wants you to be happy," and "You only live once." While each of these may sound appealing, they find their roots in tragically misguided and unbiblical philosophies.

The world's wisdom has a diabolical twin sister called the world's ways. It's a ferociously influential element that can dramatically shape us before we even realize it. There are three stand-out ways by which the world can radically renovate our mindset and cause us to drift from the ways of the Lord. They are the pressure of fitting in, the pursuit of pleasure, and the mantra "My body, my choice." While those who don't know Christ march in a trance to the hypnotic beat of the world's drums, the Christian must decide to fix his gaze on the Lord and move to the rhythm of His unalterable truth.

The man of God's greatest defense against the world's wisdom and the world's ways is in the only place where the Lord's wisdom and the Lord's ways are revealed to him—in the pages of God's inspired, infallible, and inerrant Word. Knowing the Word, being influenced by the Word, and obeying the Word will provide both a robust defense and a lethal offense. Along with that, every disciple of Christ must resist the temptation to indiscriminately immerse himself in the multiple media platforms through which the world dispenses the foolish mantras of its pseudo-wisdom. And to resist being overwhelmed and impacted by its ways, the man of God must stop focusing his mind's camera lens in on the world, but he should instead zoom out and look at everything on this planet from God's eternal perspective.

The Six Cs

Since we predominantly fight the war for sexual purity on the battlefield of our minds, victory will be determined by whether or not we choose to fight biblically in all the ways that we've already examined. A big part of our fighting strategy, therefore, must include bringing every thought into captivity to the obedience of Christ (2 Corinthians 10:5), determining to have the mind of Christ (1 Corinthians 2:16), and choosing not to be conformed to this world but instead to be transformed by the renewing of our mind (Romans 12:2). This will require both an immersion in truth and a battle plan to summon and activate that truth in a preventative, offensive, and defensive way.

In our aim to be proactively and deliberately ready to take both shield and sword in hand through having a defensive and offensive strategy against sexual temptations, our minds must be strategically prepared, and our hearts must be filled with biblical truths to draw on. Having good defensive and offensive capabilities leads to preventative preparedness, which will deter attacks from happening in the first place.

To arm us with both shield and sword and to make our defensive and offensive capabilities so robust that our enemies are deterred from even attacking us, there are six powerful truths for us to deeply understand, diligently internalize, and daily meditate on.

Creation

Sexual sin should become utterly repugnant to us when we consider the mind-blowing features and faculties that we use when engaging in it. The gateway to adultery, fornication, and masturbation is always lust. The word *creation* should remind you of the marvels of vision, cognition, and coition—elements that make lust possible. While recognizing these elements should evoke worship in our hearts, instead we often use them as instruments through which to indulge in sin and thereby harm others, ourselves, and the Lord's glory. Declare to yourself, *Creation: wield wonders as wellsprings for worship, not weapons for wounding.*

Cross

Although the cross has come to symbolize different things to different people, we know that the real cross most certainly was never meant to be a fashion accessory or a good luck charm. While it is foolishness to the world, to the Christian, the cross is the power of God unto salvation—which should make it everything to him.

As believers, consider the fact that we are called to walk in a manner that's worthy of the gospel (Philippians 1:27), which has the cross at the very center of it (1 Corinthians 15:1–3). We understand that our battle against sexual sin must be a cross-empowered and a cross-centered one. We realize that we should no longer live for ourselves but for Him who died for us on the cross before rising again (2 Corinthians 5:15). We seek to heed our Savior's call to deny ourselves, take up our cross, and follow Him. And we know that when we choose to indulge in sexual immorality, we are doing it in the very shadow of the cross. In consideration of these sobering realities, guard your steps by proclaiming to yourself, *Cross: stop spitting and stomping on such a sacred symbol.*

Crisis

Christians typically understand that crises are common occurrences in a fallen and broken world. However, the critical mistake we often make is ignoring the serious ramifications that result from them. That leads to a dangerous element of complacency, which leaves us thinking that we are not likely to do the sorts of things that would cause crises to arise in our lives.

This is a tragic error that the believer must avoid at all costs. We can sadly turn to an abundance of examples of crises related to sexual sin in the lives of others. The wise Christian will contemplate these and determine to learn from them, using this knowledge as a deterrent to sexual sin in their own life.

We also can't overlook the destruction of conscience, moral authority, leadership capacity, witness, and joy in someone experiencing the crisis of sinful choices. If ever consideration in the face of sexual pitfalls were crucial, it is certainly here. Therefore, determine to remain sober by exclaiming to yourself, *Crisis: consider the catastrophic consequences of compromise.*

Crown

In the process of discovering that eternal rewards are biblical, we learned that it's legitimate for God's children to desire them. God's rewards are far more valuable and important than anything the world could offer. The Lord makes it clear to His people that the primary foundation of faith— the type of faith that's pleasing to Him—includes not only trusting that He exists but also believing that He rewards those who diligently seek

Him (Hebrews 11:6). Jeremiah 29:12–13 reveals to us that this type of seeking after the Lord is grounded in wholeheartedness and rooted in total and glad obedience to Him. James 1:12 tells us that the Lord will give the crown of life to those who endure temptations. We also understand that this is not related to our salvation but rather precious rewards that are connected to our faithfulness to Him.

Of course, we don't know exactly what these eternal rewards will be, but we know the heart and character of the one who dispenses them. That should be enough to know that they are exceedingly good and to cause excitement to well up in our hearts when we think of them. Therefore, when we are bombarded by sexual temptations, we need to remind ourselves that this vexing crucible is very short-lived. In contrast to this transient season, our freedom will be eternal, and our choice to endure our temptations now will secure for us priceless and everlasting rewards. We top this all off by saying to ourselves, *Crown: envision endurance ensuring eternal enrichment.*

Crowd

Egocentricity seems to be everyone's favorite pet sin. Who could argue that it's not a very blinding and self-deceiving one? As it impairs our sense of reason, it simultaneously causes us to forget that the sinful decisions we make in life impact everyone within our sphere of influence. Egocentricity also makes us self-absorbed to the point of ignoring the powerful examples of the godly Christians who went before us.

When calling us to run with endurance the race that's set before us, the author of Hebrews tells us to lay aside the weights and the sin that so easily ensnare us because we are surrounded by a great cloud (or crowd) of witnesses (Hebrews 12:1). These are the saints from the great Hall of Faith who are described in Hebrews 11. These are the ones who reveled in triumphant victories and who persevered amid great trials of suffering. But all of them—despite their particular set of circumstances—have "obtained a good testimony" through faith (vv. 1–2). We see certain believers still living who are examples to us, such as Joni Eareckson Tada and many others.

By the same token, we recognize the massive impact that our decisions have on others, and this helps us realize how important it is to meditate on the crowd of witnesses who left us a powerful model to follow. We allow our minds to fixate on the faces of our wife, children, parents, siblings, nieces, nephews, aunts, uncles, cousins, neighbors, employers, employees, coworkers, mentors, mentees, friends, and others, and we cry out to ourselves with determination, *Crowd: do as the departed did and don't dispense devastation.*

Christ

It should be no wonder to us that everything for the Christian begins and ends with Jesus. After the writer of Hebrews told us to lay aside every weight and the sin that so easily ensnares us and to run with endurance the race set before us, he wrote that we should look unto Jesus, "the author and finisher of our faith" (Hebrews 12:1–2). He is, after all, "the Alpha and the Omega, the Beginning and the End, the First and the Last" (Revelation 22:13). Remembering that apart from Jesus we can do nothing (John 15:5), we look to Him as the source of supply of all that we need to have victory over sexual sin.

Most importantly, we call to mind His heart of unwavering love toward us and the fact that He is our High Priest who sympathizes with our weaknesses and who calls us to come boldly to His throne of grace in order to receive His divine help in our time of need. He can do this because He was made like us in all things except for our sinful nature, and He can therefore come to our aid whenever we're tempted (Hebrews 2:17–18).

Having such a Savior who doesn't break a bruised reed or snuff out smoking flax (Matthew 12:20–21), we should make it our aim to flee from sexual sin and walk in a manner that is worthy of Him—the one who redeemed us with His precious, priceless blood (1 Peter 1:17–19). Though we've never seen His face or heard His voice, we still rejoice over Him with joy inexpressible and full of glory, loving Him above all else because He has touched our lives like no other.

We recognize that Jesus, as the Bread of Life, is the ultimate satisfaction for our spiritual appetites—most notably for a first-love relationship, friendship, treasure, and pleasure. When we cease to feast on Christ in order to satisfy all those cravings, we end up reverting to substitution with the physical as the different stages of starvation kick in: deprivation, desperation, deviation, and deterioration. No matter how far we may stray, like the father of the prodigal son, He's always there to welcome us back home, where we can turn from the pig slop of the world's poisonous junk food and once again feast at the banqueting table of His endless love.

While the apostle John told us that we are to avoid sinning, if we do sin, Jesus is our Advocate, the one who is the propitiation for our sin (1 John 2:1–2), the one who nailed to His cross the decrees of judgment against us (Colossians 2:13–14), and the one who will never condemn us (Romans 8:1). So while you passionately pursue a life of purity, keep Jesus at the heart of your pursuit as you regularly herald to yourself, *Christ: seek the sweet Savior for strength, satisfaction, and sympathetic support.*

NOPE

Peeking, whether with our physical eyes or our mind's eye, is often the doorway to the destructive world of sexual immorality. Just one glance can put you on the precipice of a leering stare, which will inevitably thrust you headlong into the abyss of sinful lust. And if there is anything we should know about ourselves as men, it's that we are experts at justifying the unwise entertainment of sensual imagery in our hearts. The long and winding road of life will be lined with countless lust traps at every turn. What you choose to do with your eyes will determine the difference between a life of constant slavery and one of exhilarating freedom.

The old saying rings true: "You'll always be who you've always been if you always do what you've always done." A radical change in your conduct is indispensable for achieving victory. One tested strategy you can employ in your attempt to pursue radical change is to verbally exclaim, "NOPE!" whenever you're tempted to peek at any impure image that would evoke lust in you. Again, this applies whether that peek is with your physical eyes or your mind's eye. Think of the word *nope* as an acrostic that stands for "Not One Peek Even." Allow the emphatic attitude associated with this edgy declaration to strengthen your resolve to say no to lust.

It's crucial that you guard against a frantic and anxious approach to this and maintain a calm that causes you to rest in the Lord, turn away from the bait that's dangling before your eyes, and implement your predetermined battle plan. The aim is to deprive your mind and flesh of feeding on the type of lust-inducing imagery that will lead to your downfall. It's true, as Martin Luther put it, that you can't keep a bird from flying over your head, but you can keep it from nesting in your hair. If you choose to make this approach a regular practice, *NOPE* will automatically echo in the corridors of your mind and influence you to do what's right when you're faced with temptations.

May you follow in the footsteps of Job, who made a covenant with his eyes not to look lustfully at women (Job 31:1). No matter the circumstance or the setting, and whether you say it in the quietness of your mind or you proclaim it in a whisper or a shout, whenever you're tempted to peek impurely, declare to yourself, *NOPE! NOPE! NOPE! Not now. Not ever. Not One Peek Even!*

A Final Word

In nine hundred quadrillion years from now, when you're continuing to sweetly bask in the inexplicable beauty of God's eternal presence—as though you had just begun—what sinful sexual pleasure will you miss or long for? It may sound like a silly question because the answer is a given. But there's a reason why I'm asking a question that I realize you know the answer to. It's to remind you of the utter foolishness of allowing yourself to be ensnared, for even one second, by the frivolities of this fading world, especially when you're an heir to the ineffable splendor that awaits you in eternity.

Remember, you are no mere man. You will rule and reign with the conquering Christ, joining Him in judging the world and angels, reveling in every spiritual blessing with which He has blessed you in the heavenly places, and shining as a trophy of His redeeming grace as you forever display the wonders of the glorious gospel that saved you, sanctified you, and sustained you. Now that's a victory worth fighting *from*, and the glory of your amazing God is a glory worth fighting *for*. So fight tenaciously, brother. Fight courageously. Fight relentlessly. Fight in the power that He faithfully and abundantly supplies. Fight! Fight like a man!

AUTHOR'S NOTE

While the author will not be able to respond to every email, he welcomes your thoughts and feedback on *Fight Like a Man*, and he would especially love to hear the story of how the book may have impacted your life. Please send all emails to fightlikeamanfeedback@gmail.com.

If you'd like to invite the author to speak at a conference, retreat, or church service, please send your request to fightlikeamanspeaking request@gmail.com.

If you'd like to learn about the author's ministry and hear him on *The Living Waters Podcast* (one of the top-rated podcasts in the world), please visit LivingWaters.com.

ABOUT THE AUTHOR

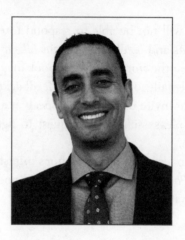

Emeal "E.Z." Zwayne is the president of Living Waters, the spokesman and host for the National Bible Bee Competition, and a cohost of *The Living Waters Podcast*. He serves as an executive producer of the *Way of the Master* television program and multiple Living Waters films. A passionate communicator, he speaks at conferences and churches nationally and around the world. E.Z. served as an associate pastor for several years. He and his wife, Rachel, have five children.